NEUTROPHIL GELATINASE-ASSOCIATED LIPOCALIN

FROM LABORATORY TO CLINICAL UTILITY

RENAL AND UROLOGIC DISORDERS

Additional books in this series can be found on Nova's website under the Series tab.

Additional e-books in this series can be found on Nova's website under the e-book tab.

NEUTROPHIL GELATINASE-ASSOCIATED LIPOCALIN

FROM LABORATORY TO CLINICAL UTILITY

MINA HUR

AND

SALVATORE DI SOMMA

EDITORS

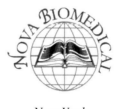

New York

For permission to use material from this book please contact us:
Telephone 631-231-7269; Fax 631-231-8175
Web Site: http://www.novapublishers.com

NOTICE TO THE READER

Library of Congress Cataloging-in-Publication Data

ISBN: 978-1-63117-984-6

Library of Congress Control Number: 2014939486

Published by Nova Science Publishers, Inc. † New York

Contents

Preface

Acute kidney injury (AKI), defined as an abrupt decrease in renal function over a period of hours to days, is a common complication especially in hospitalized patients. Currently, the diagnosis of AKI requires serial assessment of laboratory tests over a period of several days, and is based mainly on serum creatinine (sCr) as supported by Risk, Injury, Failure, Loss, and End-Stage Kidney Disease (RIFLE) criteria, Acute Kidney Injury Network (AKIN) criteria, and the recent Kidney Disease: Improving Global Outcomes (KDIGO) practice guidelines for AKI. Such a need for repeated sCr evaluations and monitoring of urinary output for several days after admission could therefore result in a delay in appropriate therapy.

As a consequence, the use of biomarkers of acute kidney damage could be of great utility in order to distinguish AKI from volume responsive renal dysfunction, chronic kidney disease (CKD), or normal renal function. Furthermore these biomarkers could contribute to the diagnosis of AKI by identifying a subgroup with 'subclinical AKI' where there may be injury even in the absence of a sCr increase, thus leading to an earlier risk stratification of patients with prompt and specific treatment strategies.

Neutrophil gelatinase-associated lipocalin (NGAL) is a relatively new biomarker for AKI. NGAL was first identified as a potential marker for AKI in 2003 through a transcriptome-wide search for genes upregulated after renal ischemia. Clinically, NGAL has got growing attention as an AKI marker, and its clinical usefulness has been investigated in a variety of clinical situations.

This specialized book is focused on lipocalin and particularly on NGAL covering the broad aspects of this biomarker from laboratory to clinical utility. This book consists of three parts: basic information on lipocalin; laboratory consideration on NGAL; and clinical utility of NGAL. Although there are many researches dealing with NGAL, this book is unique in that it is the first comprehensive book, which provides summarized and up-to-date knowledge on NGAL to the researchers and clinicians who are interested in this biomarker.

In particular, this book was conceived reflecting the spirit of GREAT network, an Academic Research Organization, operating as an International Network between experts in the management of acute diseases. Written and reviewed by the experts in each related filed, this book would be a valuable and practical reading for the researchers and clinicians working in laboratory medicine, emergency medicine, cardiology, nephrology, and intensive care, etc.

Salvatore Di Somma, M.D., Ph.D.
Professor of Medicine
Director Emergency Medicine
Chairman Postgraduate School of Emergency Medicine
Department of Medical-Surgery Sciences and Traslational Medicine
University La Sapienza Rome
Sant'Andrea Hospital;
Via di Grottarossa 1035/1039 00189 Rome (Italy)
Tel: +39 06.33775581 +39 06.33775592
Fax: +39 06.33775890
E-mail: salvatore.disomma@uniromal.it,
salvatore.disomma@ospedalesantandrea.it

Mina Hur, M.D., Ph.D.
Professor
Department of Laboratory Medicine
Konkuk University School of Medicine
Konkuk University Hospital
120-1, Neungdong-ro, Hwayang-dong
Gwangjin-gu, Seoul 143-729, Korea
Tel: +82-2-2030-5581
Fax: +82-2-2636-6764
E-mail: dearmina@hanmail.net

In: Neutrophil Gelatinase-Associated Lipocalin   ISBN: 978-1-63117-984-6
Editors: M. Hur and S. Di Somma   © 2014 Nova Science Publishers, Inc.

Chapter 1

Lipocalin: Sequence and Structure Relationships

Patrizia Cardelli[*]

Department of Molecular and Clinical Medicine,
Sant'Andrea Hospital, Sapienza University
School of Medicine, Rome, Italy

Abstract

Glycoproteins have a unique position in the pathogenesis of human diseases, playing a key role in the body's defense against diseases. Most of the commonly used protein biomarkers are glycoproteins. Examples includes cancer biomarkers like CA19-9 (carbohydrate antigen 19-9) to follow up patients with pancreatic cancer, CEA (carcinoembryonic antigen) for multiple solid tumors, and CA-125 (carbohydrate antigen 125) as well as transport proteins (retinol binding protein, a-1-acidic glycoprotein, apolipoprotein D, and apolipoprotein M). Most of these glycoproteins are large molecules but there is a family of small, secreted glycoproteins called "lipocalins", which despite a low homology of the primary structure share a similarity in the form of short characteristic conserved sequence motifs to be defined as members of a unique family. The lipocalins are fundamental in the maintenance of health and in combating diseases.

---

[*] Correspondence: patrizia.cardelli@uniroma1.it.

Introduction

Lipocalins are a large family of small (160 – 180 residues in length), with molecular masses averaging 25 kDa, phylogenetically preserved proteins occurring in bacteria, plants, and animals. Most lipocalins exhibit an N-terminal signal peptide and lack other strong hydrophobic regions, features commonly found in extracellular soluble proteins. Similarly, most lipocalins contain from one to three disulfide bridges that contribute to constraint of the overall structure by stabilizing the N- and C-terminal regions of the protein [1]. Although they have been classified mainly as transport proteins, it is now clear that members of the lipocalin family fulfill a wide variety of different functions.

Properties of Members of the Lipocalin Protein Family

Lipocalins, which are typically extracellular proteins despite the capability to bind and transport lipophilic molecules, share several common molecular recognition properties: binding to specific cell surface receptors and the formation of covalent and non-covalent complexes with other soluble macromolecules. In recent years, several additional functions have been discovered for these proteins, including regulation of cell division (e.g., α1-microglobulin), differentiation, cell-to-cell adhesion and survival (e.g., Purpurin) [2, 3]. Usually the protein family members are identified on the basis of high homologies in their amino acid sequence, but the members of the lipocalin family share much less sequence identity, in some cases as low as 20%. However, they share a common secondary and tertiary structural feature called "lipocalin fold" [3 - 6].

Structure of the Lipocalin Fold

The structure of the lipocalin protein fold is a highly symmetrical all-β structure dominated by a single eight-stranded antiparallel β-sheet closed back on itself to form a continuously hydrogen bonded β-barrel [5-7]. In cross-section, this has a flattened or elliptical shape. The β-barrel encloses a ligand binding site composed of both an internal cavity and an external loop scaffold. It is such a diversity of cavity and scaffold that gives rise to a variety of different binding modes each capable of accommodating ligands of different size, shape, and chemical character. The eight b-strands of the barrel, labeled A-H (Figure 1), are linked by a succession of +1 connections, giving it the simplest possible β-sheet topology [8]. The seven loops, labeled L1-L7, are all typical of short β-hairpins, except loop L1: this is a large β loop. Loop L1 forms a lid folded back to close partially the internal ligand-binding site found at this end of the barrel. Between strand H and the short terminal strand I is an α-helix; this is an ever-present feature of the lipocalin fold, but is not conserved in its position relative to the axis of the β-barrel nor in its length [3, 8] (Figure 1).

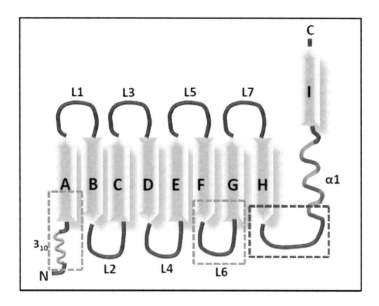

Figure 1. Schematic representation of the lipocalin fold.

The characteristic lipocalins "lipocalin fold", which comprises of an N terminal 3 - 10 helix followed by eight beta sheets (A–I) arranged in an anti-parallel orientation. The eighth beta sheet is connected to an alpha helix (denoted as α1), which is in turn connected to a C-terminal beta sheet. The beta sheets are connected by loops (L1 - L7). Loops of L1, L3, L5, and L7 form the open end of the molecule (i.e., the opening to the ligand binding site of NGAL). The portion of the lipocalin fold that are structurally conserved between different lipocalins is indicated by the blue-boxed regions, while the region that shows significant conservation in amino acid sequence is indicated by the black-boxed region. *Adapted from Chakraborty et al. [8] with permission.*

Table 1. Examples of the kernel and outlier lipocalins

Protein name	Common abbreviation	Alternative names and acronym	Molecular Weight (kDa)	Properties and Function(s)
		Kernel Lipocalins		
α1-microglobulin	α- 1M	1-m, 1m, protein HC, 1-microglycoprotein	33	Binds and degrades heme, is a radical scavenger as well as a reductase in an immunoregulator.
Apolipoprotein D	Apo-D	gross cystic disease fluid protein (GCDFP-24), apocrine secretion odourbinding protein (ASOB-2)	29–32	Member of the high density lipoprotein, Apo D has binding affinity for cholesterol, progesterone, pregnenolone, bilirubin and arachidonic acid. It is proposed to be involved in maintenance and repair of central and peripheral nervous systems.
α2-microglobulin	α -2U	rat 2-urinary globulin, mouse major urinary protein (MUP)	18.7	Abundant protein of urine and other secretions of animal, functions as pheromones, transporters of organic ions, regulators of metabolism and as potent human allergens. Major urinary protein of the male rat with extensive sequence homology to many lipid binding proteins.
Bilin binding protein	BBP	none	19.6	A blue pigment protein abundant in the butterfly *Pieris brassicae*. Binds biliverdin IXγ

Protein name	Common abbreviation	Alternative names and acronym	Molecular Weight (kDa)	Properties and Function(s)
β1-Lactoglobulin	Blg	none	18	Homolog of serum retinol-binding protein, Blg is thought to facilitate the absorption of vitamin A from milk.
subunit of human C8 complement	C8γ	none	22	As a component of the C8 complement, functions in the formation of membrane attack complex.
Choroid plexus protein	Cpl1	none	20	Proposed to transport substances across the blood brain barrier.
Retinoic acid binding protein	CRABP2	B/C protein, epididymal binding proteins 1 and 2 (EBP1/EBP2), epididymal secretory protein (ESP1), ERABP, mouse epididymal protein 10 (MEP 10)	18.3	A retinoic acid (RA) binding protein, induced by RA in RA- responsive cells and enhances transcriptional activity of RA.
α-Crustacyanin	ACC	chondrocyte 21 protein (Ch21), P20K, quiescence-speciĉc protein (QSP)	350	Responsible for the blue–black coloration of lobster carapace by causing bathochromic shifts.
Extracellular fatty acid-binding protein	Ex-FAB			Extracellular fatty acid binding
glycodelin	Glc	pregnancy protein 14 (PP14), human pregnancy-associated endometrial protein, α2 -globulin (α2-PEG),	27 - 30	Involved in implantation of the embryo and immunosuppression.

Table 1. (Continued)

Protein name	Common abbreviation	Alternative names and acronym	Molecular Weight (kDa)	Properties and Function(s)
		chorionic α2-microglobulin, progestagen associated endometrial protein (PAEP), α -uterine protein		
Neutrophil gelatinase associated Lipocalin	NGAL	human neutrophil lipocalin (HNL), 24p3, SIP24, uterocalin, α2 microglobulin-related protein, Neu-related lipocalin (NRL)	24	Discussed in text.
Prostaglandin D synthase	PGDS	β-trace	27	Involved in isomerization of Prostaglandin H2 to Prostaglandin D2.
Purpurin	PURP	none	20	Abundant protein of the neural retina, proposed to play prominent role in retinol transport across the inter-photoreceptor cell matrix.
Lazarillo	--	none	45	glycosylphosphatidyl inositol anchored surface glycoprotein, involved in the axonal growth, the regulation of lifespan, stress resistance and neuro-degeneration.
Retinol binding protein	**RBP**	**none**	**21**	**Retinol transport**

Protein name	Common abbreviation	Alternative names and acronym	Molecular Weight (kDa)	Properties and Function(s)
		Outlier Lipocalins		
α1-Acid glycoprotein	AAAG	orosomucoid (ORM), seromucoid 1 fraction, 1-S	40	Acute phase serum protein secreted by the liver in response to inflammation, stress, and various malignancies and affects pharmacokinetics of drugs.
Aphrodisin	--	None	17	A component of hamster vaginal secretions, triggers mating behavior of naive males.
Odorant binding protein	OBP	frog Bowman's gland protein	37–40	Bind to specific odorants including pheromones.
Probasin	--	pM-40	20	Androgen regulated prostate specific protein, functions as pheromone carrier.
von Ebner's-gland protein	VEGP	protein migrating faster than albumin (PMFA), specịẹc tear albumin (STP), tear lipocalin (TL), tear prealbumin(TP)	18	Salivary protein secreted by the Von Ebner's glands located around the circumvallate and foliate papilla of the human tongue, it has a large variety of ligands and secreted in response to stress, infection, and inflammation. It is suggested to inhibit cysteine proteases that are important for embryo hatching and implantation.

Adapted from [9] with permission.

Classification of Lipocalins

While the overall sequence identity between different lipocalin proteins is low, they share three regions of significant sequence and structural conservation called short conservative regions (SCR) [3]. It consists of SCR1 (strand A and the 310-like helix preceding it), SCR2 (strands F and G, and loop L6 linking them), and SCR3 (strand H and adjoining residues). Other SCRs of the common core are small and can be neglected.

The three principal SCRs each contain a sequence motif that is wholly, or partly, invariant. Lipocalins differ in their numbers of SCRs, so these regions are useful to classify all lipocalins into two broad categories: the kernel and the outlier lipocalins. While the former possess all three SCRs, the latter have only one or two, but never all three SCRs. Examples of the kernel and outlier lipocalins are summarized in Table 1 [9]. Thus, the lipocalin family is characterized by structural similarity in the absence of significant sequence identity.

Conclusion

Lipocalins are a large family of small, phylogenetically preserved proteins occurring in bacteria, plants, and animals. Although they have been classified mainly as transport proteins, members of the lipocalin family fulfill a wide variety of different functions.

Lipocalins differ in their numbers of SCRs, and classified into the kernel and the outlier lipocalins. While the former possess all three SCRs, the latter have only one or two, but never all three SCRs. The lipocalin family is characterized by structural similarity in the absence of significant sequence identity.

References

[1]   Ganfornina MD, Gutierrez D, Bastiani M, Sanchez D. A phylogenetic analysis of the lipocalin protein family. *Mol. Biol. Evol.* 2000;17:114–26.

[2]   Akerstrom B, Logdberg L, Berggard T, Osmark P, Lindqvist A. α1-
        microglobulin: a yellow-brown lipocalin. *Biochim. Biophys. Acta*
        2000;1482:172-84.

[3]   Flower DR, North ACT, Sansom CE. The lipocalin protein family:
        structural and sequence overview. *Biochim. Biophys. Acta* 2000;1482:
        9-24.

[4]   Flower DR. The lipocalin protein family: a role in cell regulation. *FEBS
        Lett.* 1994; 354:7-11.

[5]   Flower DR. Multiple molecular recognition properties of the lipocalin
        protein family. *J. Mol. Recognit.* 1995;8:185-95.

[6]   Flower DR. The lipocalin protein family: structure and function.
        Biochem. J. 1996;318:1-14.

[7]   Flower DR, North ACT, Attwood TK. Structure and sequence
        relationships in the lipocalins and related proteins. *Protein Sci.*
        1993;2:753-61.

[8]   Chakraborty S, Kaur S, Guha S, Batra SK. The multifaceted roles of
        neutrophil gelatinase-associated lipocalin (NGAL) in inflammation and
        cancer. *Biochim. Biophys. Acta 2012*;1826:129-69.

[9]   Akerstrom B, Flower DR, Salier JP. Lipocalins: unity in diversity.
        Biochim. Biophys. Acta 2000;1482:1-8.

In: Neutrophil Gelatinase-Associated Lipocalin   ISBN: 978-1-63117-984-6
Editors: M. Hur and S. Di Somma   © 2014 Nova Science Publishers, Inc.

Chapter 2

Common Molecular-Recognition Properties

Patrizia Cardelli*

Department of Molecular and Clinical Medicine,
Sant'Andrea Hospital, Sapienza University
School of Medicine, Rome, Italy

Abstract

The lipocalins display a wide range of different molecular properties, including the capacity to bind and transport small hydrophobic molecules as well as to bind to membrane surface receptors and form macromolecular complexes. This chapter provide an overview on the common molecular recognition properties of lipocalins.

Introduction

The lipocalins are known for their binding of many small hydrophobic ligands. The structure of the lipocalin fold, formed by a loop scaffold at the entrance of a large cup-shaped cavity,is well tailored to the task of ligand binding and in determining the appropriate selectivity [1,2]. To accommodate

---

* Correspondence: patrizia.cardelli@uniroma1.it.

ligands of different size and shape, the binding sites of different lipocalins can be quite different. Lipocalins bind hydrophobic ligands with a range of size and shape namely the binding of a small ligand, entirely enclosed within the internal pocket, and the binding of a large steroid, bound partly in the pocket and partly by the loop scaffold in an altogether more exposed manner [3]. For example, the binding mode of MUP, which binds its small ligand deep within its pocket entirely enclosed by side chains[4,5] can be compared with that of BBP, which binds its large and relatively hydrophilic ligand in a solvent-exposed site predominantly formed from the loop scaffold [6] (Figure 1).

Receptor or Ligand Bindings by Members of Lipocalin Protein Family

Lipocalins can complexate with soluble macromolecules by non-covalent interaction between RBP and transthyretin [7], or covalent association either by disulphide bridge (C8γ and C8α) [8], apoD and apolipoproteins [9], or NGAL and gelatinase [10], or other chemical groups (α–1M and IgA). Lipocalins can bind cell membrane receptors interacting with membrane proteins either via the lipocalin surface patch (Purpurin and C8γ) or the loop scaffold (RBP).

In the last two decades, an increasing numbers of lipocalins were found to bind to specific cell surface receptors. Some lipocalins interact with specific cell-surface receptors and release its ligand to a specific carrier protein (only the ligand is delivered inside the cell). The others are internalized as holo-lipocalins and then release their ligand inside the cells. It has been hypothesized that the three conserved sequence motifs characteristic of the family, which lie next to each other forming a surface patch at the closed end of the lipocalin fold, constitute a common cell-surface receptor binding site (Figure 1e) [11,12]. For example a cell-surface receptor for a1microglobulin (α–1M) has been identified [13,14], and there is additional evidence to suggest the existence of receptors for MUP [15,16], Blg [17,18], and OBP [19].

Epidydimal secretory protein has been shown to bindto the plasma membrane of spermatozoa and maybe another lipocalin to act via a specific surface receptor (Figure 1.d) [20,21]. An example of a lipocalin that is not internalized in the cell is RBP, which is one of the most understood lipocalin in terms of structure. Sivaprasadarao et al. [22] showed, using mutagenesis, that specific amino acids within the open end loop scaffold are responsible for binding to the RBP receptor. Recently, Redondo et al. [23] proposed that RBP binds to a specific membrane receptor and remains external to the cell, only retinol being transferred by the RBP receptor to an apo-cellular-RBP. NGAL is an example of an internalized lipocalin.

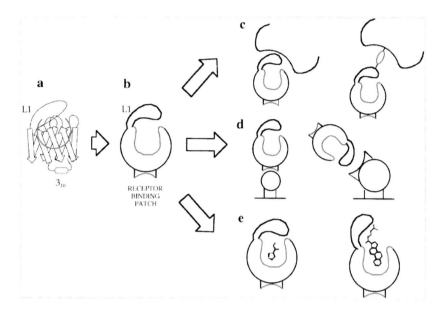

Figure 1. Polarity of the lipocalin fold and its multiple molecular recognition properties.

This figure shows a schematic representation of the lipocalin fold and visualization of the multiple interactions underlying its molecular-recognition properties. (a) Simplified schematic of the three dimensional structure of the lipocalin fold; the b-strands of the lipocalin barrel are shown as arrows; the loops of the open end of the fold are also shown, as is the N-terminal 310 helix. The location of the internal ligand-binding pocket is shown as a highlighted semicircle. (b) Highly schematic cartoon summarizing the key structural features of the lipocalin fold and emphasizing its structural polarity; the ligand-binding pocket and hypothetical receptor-binding surface patch are highlighted. (c) Complexation with soluble macromolecules. The two modes exhibited by the lipocalins are shown; non-covalent association, such as between RBP and transthyretin, and covalently linked, either by disulphides (C8c and C8a, apoD and apolipoproteins, or NGAL and gelatinase) or other groups (A1M and IgA). (d) Cell membrane receptor binding. Interaction with membrane proteins either via the lipocalin surface patch (Purpurin, C8c, etc.) or the loop scaffold (RBP). (e)Ligand-binding modes. Lipocalins bind hydrophobic ligands with a range of size and shape; extreme examples are shown, namely the binding of a small ligand, entirely enclosed within the internal pocket, and the binding of a large steroid, bound partly in the pocket and partly by the loop scaffold in an altogether more exposed manner. *Reproduced with permission, from [1] (Flower DR, 1996, Biochemical Journal, 418, 1-14).*

NGAL interacts on the cell membrane with specific receptors (24p3R and megalin) as a complex with iron-siderophores (Holo-NGAL). After internalization, Holo-NGAL is captured inside endosomal vesicles and transported within the cytoplasmic region, where it can release its siderophore-iron complex, thus activating iron-dependent specific pathways. The protein core may then be degraded or re-sent alone outside the cell [24].

Macromolecular Complexation

Lipocalins can form covalent or non-covalent complexes with soluble macromolecules, showing the ability to form dimers, or even higher level oligomers [25,26]. Aggregation is a way to pack as many molecules as possible into a small space – nature used this feature for proteins secreted by secretory glands. Some of these proteins (e.g., tick salivary gland protein), due to their β-barrel shape, can be packed better than globular proteins. Their aggregation occurs at pH 5–6 and at high calcium concentrations [27,28].

The ability of lipocalins to form complexes with soluble macromolecules is dependent on the isoelectric point of the protein and usually occurs at low pH [27,28]. So pH and ligand presence influence oligomerization in *in vitro* as well as *in vivo* conditions. The dependence of lipocalin affinity for ligands on pH-induced structural changes was used by nature for pheromone transport and presentation. It has been reported that the pH of elephant female urine is about 8, and this pH promotes pheromone binding. On the other hand, the pH in the male sensory organs, the target for pheromones, is about 5.5 [29]. Due to pH-induced structural changes, the pheromone molecule is released from its lipocalin transporter and acts directly in the place of destination.

Ligand releasing at low pH has been also shown for human tear lipocalin (hTL) [30], bovine β-lactoglobulin [31], and other lipocalins. In plasma, about 96% of total RBP is a part of a transthyretin complex [32]. Transthyretin has a higher affinity for Holo-RBP, and this interaction is sensitive to both ionic strength and pH; the complex dissociates at low ionic strength and is stable between pH 5.0 and 9.0 [32-34]. Some lipocalins exist in monomeric forms (e.g., apolipoprotein D, lazarillo, lipocalin-type prostaglandin D synthase) [35-37]. About 80% of all plasma apolipoprotein D exists as disulphide-linked complexes predominantly with apoAII in high-density lipoproteins [1,38]. The lipocalin C8γ, is covalently linked to C8α by an inter-molecular disulphide bridge [39]. Neutrophil gelatinase- associated lipocalin (NGAL) is covalently attached to MMP9 via an intermolecular disulphide bridge (Figure 1.c).

Conclusion

The lipocalins have a wide range of different molecular properties, including the capacity to bind and transport small hydrophobic molecules as well as to bind to membrane surface receptors and form macromolecular complexes. The protein-protein interactions are mediated by the loop scaffold forming the open end of the molecule. The variability of loop length and conformation and the different amino acid composition shown by these loops may be the principal means, by which different lipocalins are able to form macromolecular complexes with high affinity and selectivity.

References

[1]   Flower DR. The lipocalin protein family: structure and function. *Biochem. J.* 1996;318:1-14.

[2]   Flower DR, North ACT, Attwood TK. Structure and sequence relationships in the lipocalins and related proteins. *Protein Sci.* 1993;2:753-61.

[3]   Flower DR. Multiple molecular recognition properties of the lipocalin protein family. *J. Mol. Recognit.* 1995;8:185-95.

[4]   Shaw PH, Held WA, Hastie MD. The gene family for major urinary proteins: expression in several secretory tissues of the mouse. *Cell.* 1983;32:755-61.

[5]   Knopf JL, Gallagher JA, Held WA. Differential, multihormonal regulation of the mouse major urinary protein gene family in the liver. *Mol. Cell. Biol.* 1983;3:2232-41.

[6]   Riley CT, Barbeau BK, Keim PS, Kezdy FJ, Heinrikson RL, Law JH. The covalent protein structure of insecticyanin, a blue biliprotein from the hemolymph of the tobacco hornworm, Manduca sexta L. *J. Biol. Chem.* 1984;259:13159-65.

[7]   Newcomer ME, Ong DE. Retinol binding protein and its interaction with transthyretin. In: Madame Curie Bioscience Database [Internet]. Bookshelf ID: NBK6223 Austin (TX): *Landes Bioscience* 2000-2013.

[8]   Chiswell B, Slade DJ, Sodetz JM. Binding of the lipocalin C8gamma to human protein C8alpha is mediated by loops located at the entrance to the C8gamma ligand binding site. *Biochim. Biophys. Acta* 2006;1764:1518-24.

[9] Morais Cabral JH, Atkins GL, Sanchez LM, Lopez-Boado YS, Lopez-Otin, C, Sawyer L. Arachidonic acid binds to apolipoprotein D: implications for the protein's function. *FEBS Lett.* 1995;366:53-6.

[10] Chakraborty S, Kaur S, Guha S, Batra SK. The multifaceted roles of neutrophil gelatinase-associated lipocalin (NGAL) in inflammation and cancer. *Biochim. Biophys. Acta* 2012;1826:129-69.

[11] Akerstrom B, Logdberg L, Berggard T, Osmark P, Lindqvist A. α1-Microglobulin: a yellow-brown lipocalin. *Biochim. Biophys. Acta* 2000;1482:172-84.

[12] North ACT. Three-dimensional arrangement of conserved amino acid residues in a superfamily of specific ligand-binding proteins. *Int. J. Biol. Macromol.* 1989;11:56-8.

[13] Akerstrom B, Logdberg L. An intriguing member of the lipocalin protein family: alpha 1-microglobulin. *Trends Biochem. Sci.* 1990;15:240-3.

[14] Magnus G, Olsson EJ, Nilsson C, Rutardóttir S, Paczesny J, Pallon J, Åkerström B. Bystander cell death and stress response is inhibited by the radical scavenger α(1)-microglobulin in irradiated cell cultures. *Radiat. Res.* 2010;174:590-600.

[15] Böcskei Z, Groom CR, Flower DR, Wright CE, Phillips SE, Cavaggioni A, Findlay JB, North AC. Pheromone binding to two rodent urinary proteins revealed by X-ray crystallography. *Nature* 1992;360:186-8.

[16] Crossett B, Allen WR, Stewart F. A 19 kDa protein secreted by the endometrium of the mare is a novel member of the lipocalin family. *Biochem J.* 1996;320:137-43.

[17] Hambling SG, McAlpine AS, and Sawyer L. In: Advanced Dairy Chemistry, (1992) 1 (Fox,PF, ed.), 140-190, *Elsevier Applied Science*, London.

[18] Mansouri A, Guéant JL, Capiaumont J, Pelosi P, Nabet P, Haertlé T. Plasma membrane receptor for beta-lactoglobulin and retinol-binding protein in murine hybridomas. *Biofactors* 1998;7:287-98.

[19] Boudjelal M, Sivaprasadarao A, Findlay JB. Membrane receptor for odour-binding proteins. *Biochem. J.* 1996;317:23-7.

[20] Morel L, Dufaure JP, Depeiges A. LESP, an androgen-regulated lizard epididymal secretory protein family identified as a new member of the lipocalin superfamily. *J. Biol. Chem.* 1993;268:10274-81.

[21] Chen DY, Liu SJ, Zhu MY, Li WY, Cui YD, Huang YF. Different expression of lipocalin-type prostaglandin D synthase in rat epididymidis. *Anim. Reprod. Sci.* 2007;98:302-10.

[22] Sivaprasadarao A, Sundaram M, Findlay JB. Interactions of retinol-binding protein with transthyretin and its receptor. *Methods Mol. Biol.* 1998;89:155-63.

[23] Redondo C, Vouropoulou M, Evans J, Findlay JB. Identification of the retinol-binding protein (RBP) interaction site and functional state of RBPs for the membrane receptor. *FASEB J.* 2008;22:1043-54.

[24] Langelueddecke C, Roussa E, Fenton RA, Wolff NA, Lee WK, Thévenod F. Lipocalin-2 (24p3/neutrophil gelatinase-associated lipocalin (NGAL)) receptor is expressed in distal nephron and mediates protein endocytosis. *J. Biol. Chem.* 2012;287:159-69.

[25] Akerstrom B, Flower DR, Salier JP. Lipocalins: unity in diversity. *Biochim. Biophys. Acta* 2000;1482:1-8.

[26] Grzyb J, Latowski D, Strzałka K. Lipocalins - a family portrait. *J. Plant. Physiol.* 2006;163:895-915.

[27] Mans BJ, Louw AI, Neitz AW. The major tick salivary gland proteins and toxins from the soft tick, Ornithodorossavignyi, are part of the tick Lipocalin family: implications for the origins of tick toxicoses. *Mol. Biol. Evol.* 2003;20:1158-67.

[28] Mans BJ, Ribeiro JM. Function, mechanism and evolution of the moubatin-clade of soft tick lipocalins. Insect Biochem. *Mol. Biol.* 2008;38:841-52.

[29] Rasmussen LEL. Source and cyclic release pattern of (Z)-7-dodecenyl acetate, the pre-ovulatory pheromone of the female Asian elephant. *Chem. Senses* 2001;26: 611–23.

[30] Dartt DA. Tear lipocalin: structure and function. *Ocul. Surf.* 2011;9:126-38.

[31] Ragona L, Pusterla F, Zetta L, Monaco HL, Molinari H. Identification of a conserved hydrophobic cluster in partially folded bovine beta-lactoglobulin at pH 2. *Fold. Des.* 1997;2:281-90.

[32] Noy N, Slosberg E, Scarlata S. Interactions of retinol with binding proteins: studies with retinol-binding protein and with transthyretin. *Biochemistry* 1992;31:11118-24.

[33] Aqvist J, Sandblom P, Jones TA, Newcomer ME, van Gunsteren WF, Tapia O. Molecular dynamics simulations of the holo and apo forms of retinol binding protein. Structural and dynamical changes induced by retinol removal. *J. Mol. Biol.* 1986;192:593-603.

[34] Zanotti G, Folli C, Cendron L, Alfieri B, Nishida SK, Gliubich F, Pasquato N, Negro A, Berni R. Structural and mutational analyses of

protein-protein interactions between transthyretin and retinol-binding protein. *FEBS J.* 2008;275:5841-54.

[35] Urade Y, Fujimoto N, Hayaishi O. Purification and characterization of rat brain prostaglandin D synthetase. *J. Biol. Chem.* 1985;260:12410–5.

[36] Peitsch MC, Boguski MS. Is apolipoprotein D a mammalian bilin-binding protein? *New Biol.* 1990;2:197–206.

[37] Sanchez D, Ganfornina MD, Bastiani MJ. Lazarillo, a neuronal lipocalin in grasshoppers with a role in axon guidance. *Biochim. Biophys. Acta* 2000;1482:102–9.

[38] Blanco-Vaca F, Via DP, Yang CY, Massey JB, Pownall HJ. Characterization of disulfide-linked heterodimers containing apolipoprotein D in human plasma lipoproteins. *J. Lipid. Res.* 1992;33:1785-96.

[39] Slade DJ, Lovelace LL, Chruszcz M, Minor W, Lebioda L, Sodetz JM. Crystal structure of the MACPF domain of human complement protein C8 alpha in complex with the C8 gamma subunit. *J. Mol. Biol.* 2008;379:331-42.

In: Neutrophil Gelatinase-Associated Lipocalin   ISBN: 978-1-63117-984-6
Editors: M. Hur and S. Di Somma   © 2014 Nova Science Publishers, Inc.

Chapter 3

Biochemistry and Pathophysiology of NGAL

Patrizia Cardelli[*]

Department of Molecular and Clinical Medicine, Sant'Andrea
Hospital, Sapienza University School of Medicine, Rome, Italy

Abstract

NGAL belongs to the lipocalin family of protein, and, in humans, it is encoded by the *LCN2* gene. It is a small secreted proteins characterized by their ability to bind small, hydrophobic molecules including sidero-phores, in a structurally conserved pocket formed by a β-pleated sheet and to form macromolecular complexes.

NGAL has a variety of functions, including the regulation of the immune response and the mediation of cell homeostasis.

Introduction

NGAL is known with many different names as 24p3, oncogene 24p3, p25, migration stimulating factor inhibitor (MSFI), neutrophil glucosaminidase-associated lipocalin, human neutrophil lipocalin (HNL), α1-microglobulin

---

[*]Corresponding author: Patrizia Cardelli. E-mail: patrizia.cardelli@uniroma1.it.

related protein, siderocalin, or uterocalin. It is a glycoprotein encoded by a gene located at the chromosome locus 9q34.11. The NGAL gene is constituted by seven exons that produce at least five functional transcripts, the most common of which encodes a 198 amino acid secreted protein. It was first isolated and purified from mouse kidney cells infected with a simian virus (SV-40) [1]. The mouse homologue of human NGAL or lipocalin 2 is represented in lower case (Lcn2 or Ngal) to distinguish it from its human counterpart (LCN2 or NGAL) [2].

NGAL was first isolated by Triebel et al. [3] as a 25 kDa glycoprotein that was associated with the monomeric form of matrix metalloproteinase-9 (MMP-9). This gelatinase secreted by neutrophils degrades several basement membranes and components of the extracellular matrix like cartilage proteoglycan, type I gelatin, and collagens type I, IV, V and XI [3]. They called it α2-microglobulin related protein (α2-MRP), because it had a sequence homology to the rat α2-microglobulin protein. The association between α2-MRP (or NGAL) and MMP-9 appeared to occur through a disulfide bond that could be broken under reducing conditions. Moreover, this association did not affect the enzymatic activity of MMP-9 against a synthetic substrate, suggesting that α2-MRP or NGAL had a role in modulating the stability rather than the enzymatic activity of MMP-9. Based on whether NGAL is free or bound to a ligand, it is termed as "apo" or "holo" NGAL, respectively. The conformational change between these two forms of protein is affected by a conformation change occurring at the open end of the NGAL protein.

Domain Structure of NGAL

The human NGAL has 98% identity to the homologue protein present in chimpanzee, showing less similarity to the mouse (62%) and rat (63%) Lcn2 homologues. Despite the limited identity of their amino acid sequences, the mouse and human homologue shares a similar domain architecture and three-dimensional structure. This feature is a characteristic of the lipocalin-family and underlies the conserved function of the lipocalin domain.

The analysis of the protein sequence of human NGAL reveals two main features, a 20 amino acid N-terminal signal peptide and a lipocalin domain (amino acids 48–193) which makes up most of the length of the molecule. The lipocalin domain (the lipocalin fold) is the characteristic feature of the lipocalin family and contains the ligand binding region that binds to and transports small lipophilic ligands (including retinoids, steroids, and iron) [4, 5].

Three Dimensional Structure of NGAL

Nuclear magnetic resonance studies showed that the NGAL molecule contains eight antiparallel β strands that form a barrel shaped structure [6]. Three β bulges present in this barrel, one formed by the 1st and two by the 6th β strand, have been suggested to contribute to the ligand binding site of NGAL. Hydrophobic residues (Trp 31, Trp 33, Val 66, Phe 83, Phe 92, Phe 94, Val 108, Val 110, Val 121, and Phe 123) present at the base of this barrel-like structure have been shown to be involved in direct binding to the ligand. On the other hand, the region closer to the opening of the barrel is comprised of polar residues (Tyr 52, Thr 54, Tyr56, Tyr 106, Thr 136, and Tyr 138). Near the mouth of the barrel, side chains of three highly polar residues (Lys 125, Lys 134, and Arg 81) project into the cup-like ligand binding cavity of NGAL.

Further, a negatively charged "pit" present at the base of the barrel formed by the amino acids aspartate and glutamate (Asp 34, Glu 60, and Asp 61) and a nearby unpaired Cysteine residue (Cys 87) has been suggested to be crucial for binding of NGAL to the gelatinase MMP-9.

The cavity in NGAL differs from that of other lipocalins in being significantly polar and it can links macromolecular ligands like proteins [7].

NGAL specifically interacts with bacterial proteins named siderophores that bind to circulating and intracellular free iron. These are low molecular weight proteins produced by microorganisms that bind to the ferric (Fe^{3+}) form of iron. Siderophores are necessary for the survival of many micro-organisms in the human body where they are exposed to iron deficiency, due to the very low circulating levels of unbound iron [8].

Siderophores have a very high affinity for free ferric iron and can bind it, making iron available to the microorganism [9]. It must be underlined that NGAL binds to iron complexed with siderophores but not to free iron [10].

Mainly NGAL can bind two classes of siderophores, the phenolate/catecholate type produced by gram-negative Enterobacteria, which are significantly polar, and carboxymycobactin (CMB) type produced by mycobacteria like *Mycobacterium tuberculosis*, which are more hydrophobic [11].

The former binds to the polar residues that make up the cup-like ligand binding pocket (of NGAL), while a different set of residues mediate the binding of the latter the more hydrophobic CMBs, which better fit into the ligand binding pocket of NGAL [11].

Accordingly, NGAL possesses "ligand plasticity" and is able to bind to a wide variety of ligand, thus mediate its physiologic role as a broad specificity "siderophore-binding protein" of the innate immune system.

Biological Activity of NGAL

The biological activity of NGAL is mediated by means of bonds with specific surface receptors, including the 24p3R, a brain-type organic cation transporter, and the megalin multiscavenger complex, mainly present on the brush-border surface of renal tubular cells [12, 13].

After interaction with these receptors, NGAL is internalized inside the cell as Holo-NGAL or as Apo-NGAL (Figure 1.3.1) [14]. Holo-NGAL is captured inside endosomal vesicles and transported within the cytoplasm, where it can release the siderophore-iron complex, thus activating iron-dependent specific pathways. Conversely, Apo-NGAL, after being internalized in the cell, is able to capture cellular iron and export it to the extracellular space (Figure 1.3.1).

This results in depletion of iron cellular pools that, under particular conditions, may even lead to apoptosis. Due to its specific binding to bacterial siderophores, NGAL is also able to exert a bacteriostatic effect on several strains of bacteria by its ability to capture siderophores in extracellular space and so to deplete the bacterial iron supply [15-17]. Therefore, NGAL represents a critical component of innate immunity to bacterial infection [17]. NGAL seems to have more complex activities than just its antimicrobial effect. Indeed, NGAL shows complex interactions with several other receptors and ligands, such as hepatocyte growth factor, some gelatinases like as matrix metalloproteinase-9 (MMP-9), and extracellular protein kinases [15, 18-20], which are involved in several biological responses, such as cell proliferation and differentiation [16].

Mechanism of Induction and Elimination of NGAL

Human NGAL was firstly isolated in the late granules of human neutrophils. NGAL mRNA is expressed in adult human tissues including the kidneys, liver, lungs, trachea, breast ducts, small intestine, bone marrow, thymus, prostate, adipose tissue, and macrophages. Low expression of NGAL is detected in pancreas, endometrial glands, thymus, and peripheral blood leucocytes, and it is absent in the brain, heart, skeletal muscle, spleen, testes, ovary, and colon [5, 21-25]. In human fetal tissues, NGAL is expressed in trophoblastic cells of the placenta, in chondrocytes, and in the epithelial cells of the developing lung and small intestine.

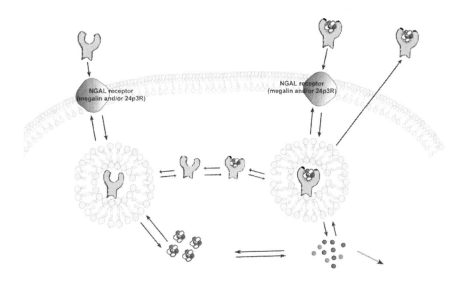

Modified from Bolignano et al. 2008. [14] with permission.

Figure 1.3.1. NGAL cellular turnover. NGAL interacts with specific receptors (24p3R or megalin) as Holo-NGAL or as Apo-NGAL. After internalization, Holo-NGAL can release the iron into the cytoplasm, leading to iron accumulation and regulating specific iron-dependent gene pathways. Then NGAL may be destroyed within the cell or recycled outside as Apo-NGAL. Conversely, Apo-NGAL can capture intracellular iron-siderophores and transport them to the extracellular space, thus depriving the cell of its iron reserves.

From the 5th month of gestation, NGAL expression has been reported in the epidermis and with increasing age of the fetus, this expression spreads to the lower layers of the skin becoming higher around the hair follicles [26]. In healthy people, human neutrophils are the main cellular source of circulating NGAL [4].

NGAL exists in different forms: a monomer of 25 kDa, a dimer of 46 kDa, and a homotrimer of 70 kDa, and as a complex with MMP-9 of 92 kDa [27, 28]. NGAL expression appears to be influenced by several molecules like cytokines, growth factors, hormones, vitamins, minerals, and synthetic drugs (Table 1) [29].

Each of these molecules probably acts in a context dependent manner to influence the expression of this glycoprotein. NF-κB, a transcription factor and regulator of several key pathways in the cell, has shown its fundamental importance in the regulation of NGAL gene expression.

Table 1. Molecules influencing NGAL expression

Family	Molecule	Effect on NGAL expression
Cytokines		
	Granulocyte monocyte colony stimulating factor (GM-CSF)	Upregulation
	Interleukin 1 alpha (IL-1α)	
	Interleukin 1 beta (IL-1β)	
	Interleukin 17 (IL-17)	
	Interleukin 22 (IL-22)	
	Transforming growth factor alpha (TGF-α)	
	Tumor necrosis factor alpha (TNF-α)	None/downregulation
	Interleukin 6 (IL-6)	None
	Basic fibroblast growth factor (bFGF)	
Growth factors		
	Insulin like growth factor-1 (IGF-1)	Upregulation
	Epidermal growth factor (EGF)	Up/downregulation
Synthetic drugs		
	Synthetic corticosteroid dexamethasone	Upregulation
	Iron-chelator deferoxamine	
	Synthetic nonsteroidal estrogen diethylstilbestrol	
	Demethylating agent 5-azacytidine	
Hormones		
	Insulin	Upregulation
	Estrogen	Up/downregulation
	Progesterone	None
Bacterial components		
	Lipopolysaccharide (TLR-4 ligand) LPS	Upregulation

Family	Molecule	Effect on NGAL expression
	Gram positive bacterial cell wall components Lipotechoic acid, Peptidoglycan	
TLRs ligands		
	Pam3CSK4 (TLR-1/2)	Upregulation
	Flagellin (TLR-5) l	
	Polyinosinic polycytidylic acid (TLR-3)	
	Unmethylated CpG oligonucleotides (TLR-9 ligand)	

Moreover, NGAL has been shown to be positively regulated by molecules that induce NF-κB, such as insulin, IL-1β, and TLRs. A second pathway that has been shown to promote NGAL expression is the JNK (c-Jun N-terminal kinase) MAPK pathway.

Cytokines like IL-1 and IL-17 can both activate the JNK pathway. A crosstalk between the JNK and NF-κB has been suggested to act together to upregulate NGAL expression [30-32].

Because of its small molecular size and resistance to degradation, NGAL is readily excreted and detected in the urine, both in its free form and in complex with MMP-9. Urinary levels correlate with plasma or serum levels whatever the cause of increased NGAL production, but high urinary levels can be expected when it is released directly into the urine by the kidney tubules. It is uncertain how far NGAL-MMP-9 complexes from sources remote from the urinary tract are excreted as such into the urine or reform in the urine after independent excretion of NGAL and MMP-9 [33].

So, circulating NGAL concentration is the result of a complex cell/tissue expression modulated by a relatively small number of pathways, which can be up- or down-regulated in dependence of different pathological conditions.

Conclusion

NGAL can be present in two forms: Apo-NGAL and Holo-NGAL. The conformational change between these two forms of protein is affected by a conformation change occurring at the open end of the NGAL protein.

The lipocalin fold is the characteristic feature of the lipocalin family and contains the ligand binding region that binds to and transports small lipophilic ligands.

NGAL specifically interacts with bacterial proteins named siderophores that bind to circulating and intracellular free iron. In addition to its antimicrobial effect, NGAL seems to have more complex activities involved in several biological responses, such as cell proliferation and differentiation.

Human neutrophils are the main cellular source of circulating NGAL, and NGAL is readily excreted and detected in the urine, both in its free form and in complex with MMP-9.

References

[1]   Hraba-Renevey, S., Turler, H., Kress, M., Salomon, C., Weil, R. SV40-induced expression of mouse gene 243 involves a post-transcriptional mechanism. *Oncogene* 1989;4:601-8.

[2]   Kjeldsen, L., Cowland, J. B., Borregaard, N. Human neutrophil gelatinse-associated lipocalin and homologous proteins in rat and mouse. *Biochim. Biophys. Acta* 2000;1482:272–83.

[3]   Triebel, S., Blaser, J., Reinke, H., Tschesche, H. A 25 kDa alpha 2-microglobulin-related protein is a component of the 125 kDa form of human gelatinase. *FEBS Lett.* 1992;314:386–8.

[4]   Chakraborty, S., Kaur, S., Guha, S., Batra, S. K. The multifaceted roles of neutrophil gelatinase associated lipocalin (NGAL) in inflammation and cancer. *Biochim. Biophys. Acta* 2012;1826:129-69.

[5]   Cowland, J. B., Borregaard, N. Molecular characterization and pattern of tissue expression of the gene for neutrophil gelatinase-associated lipocalin from humans. *Genomics* 1997;45:17-23.

[6]   Coles, M., Diercks, T., Muehlenweg, B., Bartsch, S., Zolzer, V., Tschesche, H., Kessler, H. The solution structure and dynamics of human neutrophil gelatinase-associated lipocalin. *J. Mol. Biol.* 1999; 289:139–57.

[7]   Goetz, D. H., Willie, S. T., Armen, R. S., Bratt, T., Borregaard, N., Strong, R. K. Ligand preference inferred from the structure of neutrophil gelatinase associated lipocalin. *Biochemistry* 2000;39:1935–41.

[8]   Payne, S. M., Finkelstein, R. A. The critical role of iron in host-bacterial interactions. *J. Clin. Invest.* 1978;61:1428–40.

[9]   Neilands, J. B. Siderophores: structure and function of microbial iron transport compounds. *J. Biol. Chem.* 1995;270:26723–6.

[10]   Goetz, D. H., Holmes, M. A., Borregaard, N., Bluhm, M. E., Raymond, K. N., Strong, R. K. The neutrophil lipocalin NGAL is a bacteriostatic

agent that interferes with siderophore-mediated iron acquisition. *Mol. Cell* 2002;10:1033–43.

[11]   Holmes, M. A., Paulsene, W., Jide, X., Ratledge, C., Strong, R. K. Siderocalin (Lcn 2) also binds carboxymycobactins, potentially defending against mycobacterial infections through iron sequestration. *Structure* 2005;13:29–41.

[12]   Devireddy, L. R., Gazin, C., Zhu, X., Green, M. R. A cell surface receptor for lipocalin 24p3 selectively mediates apoptosis and iron uptake. *Cell* 2005;123:1293–305.

[13]   Hvidberg, V., Jacobsen, C., Strong, R. K., Cowland, J. B., Moestrup, S. K., Borregaard, N. The endocytic receptor megalin binds the iron transporting neutrophil-gelatinase-associated lipocalin with high affinity and mediates its cellular uptake. *FEBS Lett.* 2005;579:773–7.

[14]   Bolignano, D., Donato, V., Coppolino, G., Campo, S., Buemi, A., Lacquaniti, A., Buemi, M. Neutrophil gelatinase-associated lipocalin (NGAL) as a marker of kidney damage. *Am. J. Kidney Dis.* 2008;52: 595-605.

[15]   Clifton, M. C., Corrent, C., Strong, R. K. Siderocalins: siderophore binding proteins of the innate immune system. *Biometals* 2009;22:557–64.

[16]   Schmidt-Ott, K. M., Mori, K., Li, J. Y., Kalandadze, A., Cohen, D. J., Devarajan, P., Barasch, J. Dual action of neutrophil gelatinase-associated lipocalin. *J. Am. Soc. Nephrol.* 2007;18:407–13.

[17]   Flo, T. H., Smith, K. D., Sato, S., Rodriguez, D. J., Holmes, M. A., Strong, R. K., Akira, S., Aderem, A. Lipocalin 2 mediates an innate immune response to bacterial infection by sequestrating iron. *Nature* 2004;432:917–21.

[18]   Flower, D. R., North, A. C., Attwood, T. K. Structure and sequence relationships in the lipocalins and related proteins. *Protein Sci.* 1993; 2: 753-61.

[19]   Devarajan, P. Neutrophil gelatinase-associated lipocalin: a promising biomarker for human acute kidney injury. *Biomarkers Med.* 2010;4:265–80.

[20]   Borregaard, N., Cowland, J. B. Neutrophil gelatinase-associated lipocalin, a siderophore-binding eukaryotic protein. *Biometals* 2006;19: 211–5.

[21]   Le Cabec, V., Calafat, J., Borregaard, N. Sorting of the specific granule protein, NGAL, during granulocytic maturation of HL-60 cells. *Blood* 1997;89:2113-21.

[22] Seth, P., Porter, D., Lahti-Domenici, J., Geng, Y., Richardson, A., Polyak, K. Cellular and molecular targets of estrogen in normal human breast tissue. *Cancer Res.* 2002;62:4540-4.

[23] Moreno-Navarrete, J. M., Manco, M., Ibanez, J., Garcia-Fuentes, E., Ortega, F., Gorostiaga, E., Vendrell, J., Izquierdo, M., Martinez, C., Nolfe, G., Ricart, W., Mingrone, G., Tinahones, F., Fernandez-Real, J. M. Metabolic endotoxemia and saturated fat contribute to circulating NGAL concentrations in subjects with insulin resistance. *Int. J. Obes.* (Lond.) 2010;34:240-9.

[24] Furutani, M., Arii, S., Mizumoto, M., Kato, M., Imamura, M. Identification of a neutrophil gelatinase-associated lipocalin mRNA in human pancreatic cancers using a modified signal sequence trap method. *Cancer Lett.* 1998;122: 209-14.

[25] Cowland, J. B., Sorensen, M., Sehested, N., Borregaard, N. Neutrophil gelatinase-associated lipocalin is up-regulated in human epithelial cells by IL-1 beta, but not by TNF-alpha. *J. Immunol.* 2003;171:6630-9.

[26] Mallbris, L., O'Brien, K. P., Hulthen, A., Sandstedt, B., Cowland, J. B., Borregaard, N., Stahle-Backdahl, M. Neutrophil gelatinase-associated lipocalin is a marker for dysregulated keratinocyte differentiation in human skin. *Exp. Dermatol.* 2002;11:584-91.

[27] Axelsson, L., Bergenfeldt, M., Ohlsson, K. Studies of the release and turnover of a human neutrophil lipocalin. *Scand. J. Clin. Lab. Invest.* 1995;55:577–88.

[28] Provatopoulou, X., Gounaris, A., Kalogera, E., Zagouri, F., Flessas, I., Goussetis, E., Nonni, A., Papassotiriou, I., Zografos, G. Circulating levels of matrix metalloproteinase-9 (MMP-9), neutrophil gelatinase-associated lipocalin (NGAL) and their complex MMP-9/NGAL in breast cancer disease. *BMC Cancer* 2009;9:390.

[29] Chakraborty, S., Kaur, S., Tong, Z., Batra, S. K., Guha, S. (2011). Neutrophil Gelatinase Associated Lipocalin: Structure, Function and Role in Human Pathogenesis, *Acute Phase Proteins - Regulation and Functions of Acute Phase Proteins*, Prof. Francisco Veas (Ed.), ISBN: 978-953-307-252-4, InTech, DOI: 10.5772/18755. Available from: http://www.intechopen.com/books/acute-phase-proteins-regulation-and-functions-of-acute-phase-proteins/neutrophil-gelatinase-associated-lipocalin-structure-function-and-role-in-human-pathogenesis.

[30] Florin, L., Hummerich, L., Dittrich, B. T., Kokocinski, F., Wrobel, G., Gack, S., Schorpp-Kistner, M., Werner, S., Hahn, M., Lichter, P., Szabowski, S., Angel, P. Identification of novel AP-1 target genes in

fibroblasts regulated during cutaneous wound healing. *Oncogene* 2004; 23:7005-17.

[31] Yang, X. O., Chang, S. H., Park, H., Nurieva, R., Shah, B., Acero, L., Wang, Y. H., Schluns, K. S., Broaddus, R. R., Zhu, Z., Dong, C. Regulation of inflammatory responses by IL-17F. *J. Exp. Med.* 2008; 205:1063-75.

[32] Park, H., Li, Z., Yang, X. O., Chang, S. H., Nurieva, R., Wang, Y. H., Wang, Y., Hood, L., Zhu, Z., Tian, Q., Dong, C. A distinct lineage of CD4 T cells regulates tissue inflammation by producing interleukin 17. *Nat. Immunol.* 2005;6:1133-41.

[33] Yan, L., Borregaard, N., Kjeldsen, L., Moses, M. A. The high molecular weight urinary matrix metalloproteinase (MMP) activity is a complex of gelatinase B/MMP-9 and neutrophil gelatinase-associated lipocalin (NGAL). Modulation of MMP-9 activity by NGAL. *J. Biol. Chem.* 2001; 276:37258-65.

In: Neutrophil Gelatinase-Associated Lipocalin   ISBN: 978-1-63117-984-6
Editors: M. Hur and S. Di Somma   © 2014 Nova Science Publishers, Inc.

Chapter 4

Function of Lipocalin

Patrizia Cardelli[*]
Department of Molecular and Clinical Medicine, Sant'Andrea
Hospital, Sapienza University, School of Medicine,
Rome, Italy

Abstract

The lipocalins are a family of extracellular proteins that bind and transport small hydrophobic molecules and participate in the distribution/ delivery of these substances. They are found in bacteria and in a great variety of eukaryotic cells, in which they play diverse physiological roles. They play an important role in the regulation of immunological and developmental processes, and are involved in the reactions of organisms to various stress factors and in the pathways of signal transduction. Furthermore, a few members of the lipocalin family showed enzymatic activity, as well as the capacity to interact with natural membranes, both directly with the phospholipid bilayer and/or through membrane bound receptors.

[*] Corresponding author: Patrizia Cardelli. E-mail: patrizia.cardelli@uniroma1.it.

Introduction

The lipocalin family exhibits a variety of physiological roles. Some proteins in the lipocalin family, immunocalins, are involved in immune and inflammatory response, showing immunoregulatory, antinflammatory, and antimicrobial effects. The other lipocalins scavenge for potentially toxic and harmful molecules and bind and transport metals such as iron that is essential for all organisms' life. Most mammal-derived respiratory allergens, as well as a milk allergens and few insect allergens, belong to the lipocalin protein family.

The lipocalin family is also involved in the transport of mammalian pheromones, prostaglandin (PG) synthesis, and retinol binding.

Immune and Inflammatory Response

The plasma levels of some proteins are modified during the acute phase response to local or systemic inflammation in many disease states. At least seven of these proteins belong to the lipocalin family and are identified as immunocalins. Five of them have been reported to be positive acute phase proteins (APPs). These immunocalins are alpha-1-acid glycoprotein (AGP) [1], alpha-1-microglobulin (1M) [2, 3], glycodelin (Gd) [4], neutrophil gelatinase-associated protein (NGAL) [5], and the complement factor C8-subunit (C8G) [6].

Several of them are not traditional positive APPs, but it is remarkable that all five are members of the same subset of lipocalins that are encoded by a cluster of genes in the q32-34 region of chromosome 9 in the human genome.

This cluster includes the genes for at least two other members of the lipocalin family: tear prealbumin (TP) [7] and lipocalin prostaglandin D synthase (LPGDS) [8].

It is remarkable that all seven of these lipocalins exhibit protective immunoregulatory, antinflammatory, and antimicrobial effects.

Cellular Detoxification

Some lipocalins can act as cellular nano-cleaners. They scavenge for potentially toxic and harmful molecules and bind and transport metals such as iron which is essential for all organisms' life. Bacteria and prokaryotic cells use iron-chelating molecules called siderophores to exploit this element from eukaryotic organisms. Otherwise, eukaryotic cells developed special lipocalins called siderocalins, which are able to pick up bacterial siderophores and thus prevent bacterial growth [9-11].

With respect to their protective role, lipocalins can be characterized on the basis of their affinity for a particular type of ligand. One group of lipocalins primarily binds siderophores, such as iron-binding lipocalin 2 also called siderocalin or NGAL [9, 12, 13] and lipocalin 1 also called human tear lipocalin [13]. A second group of lipocalins that possess a smaller beta barrels have no capacity to bind siderophores, but their scavenger role involves binding of ligands connected to reactive oxygen species.

Efficiency of such a ligand binding by lipocalins varies widely throughout the spectrum of all described lipocalins, including lipocalins from bacteria, plants, insects, and mammals [14, 15].

Allergens

Most mammal-derived respiratory allergens, as well as a milk allergens and few insect allergens, belong to the lipocalin protein family. Mammalian lipocalin allergens are ubiquitous present in the indoor environments.

Lipocalin allergens do not exhibit any known physicochemical, functional, or structural property that would account for their allergenicity, that is, the capacity to induce T-helper type 2 immunity against them [16].

A distinctive feature of mammalian lipocalin allergens is their poor capacity to stimulate the cellular immune system.

Nevertheless, they induce IgE production in a large proportion of atopic individuals exposed to the allergen source. The poor capacity of mammalian lipocalin allergens to stimulate the cellular immune system does not appear to result from the function of regulatory T cells. Instead, the T cell epitopes of mammalian lipocalin allergens are few and those examined have proved to be suboptimal. Moreover, the frequency of mammalian lipocalin allergen-specific CD4 (+) T cells is very low in the peripheral blood.

Importantly, recent research suggests that the lipocalin allergen-specific T cell repertoires differ considerably between allergic and healthy subjects. Several lipocalins exhibit homologies of 40-60% over species.

Mammalian lipocalin allergens may be immunologically at the borderline between self and non-self, which would not allow a strong anti-allergenic immune response against them [17].

Pheromone and Odorant Transport

The lipocalin family is involved in the transport of mammalian pheromones [18]. In the liver, volatile ligands like pheromones are encapsulated by secretory lipocalins which are released in the blood and then via glomerular filtration are excreted out of the body. In salivary glands, pheromones are encapsulated by lipocalins and secreted into oral cavity, and then these proteins can be spread onto the mammals' fur where they dry and release pheromones.

The activity of pheromones that enter the nasal cavity during breathing may be prolonged by salivary and nasal lipocalins. These pheromone-lipocalin complexes are likely to be consecutively passed to the proximity of chemosensory neurons, where they cause prolonged or more intense signal transduction when pheromones bind to an extra-cellular part of G-protein coupled receptors. Then, the pheromone-lipocalin complexes can pass the information from chemosensory neurons to central nervous system (CNS) via long axons [18].

Another group of lipocalins involved in chemical communication includes odorant binding proteins (Obp). So far, various Obp-like sequences were reported from different mammalian species including humans [19]. It must be emphasized that there is neither clear border between odorants and pheromones nor the evidence that specific pheromone binding lipocalins specifically bind only pheromones and not odorants. They are involved: (i) in the transport of odorants to the olfactory receptors [20]; (ii) in facilitating the transfer of ligands to the olfactory receptors from ligand-Obp complexes; (iii) to act as deactivators by removing the odorants from the olfactory receptors and also scavenge for potentially cytotoxic and genotoxic compounds.

Furthermore, the role of Obp may yield a prolongation of the activity of given signal by a prolonged retention and consecutive release of ligands that are encapsulated by these proteins [21]. Such mechanisms may be essential in the amplification of the output signal of olfactory neurons in the brain.

Prostaglandin Synthesis

Lipocalin-type prostaglandin (PG) D synthase (L-PGDS) or β–trace was first described as a major protein of cerebrospinal fluid [22], where it catalyze the isomerization of PG H2 (PGH2) to PG D2 (PGD2), the major prostanoid produced in the CNS of mammals [23].

It is a bifunctional protein that possesses both the ability to synthesize PGD2 and to serve as a carrier protein for lipophilic molecules; moreover, it is the only enzyme among the members of lipocalin protein family [24].

Prostaglandin D synthase (PGDS) is an enzyme involved in the metabolism of arachidonic acid and is responsible for the conversion of PGH2 to PGD2. The levels of PGD2 and its metabolites are elevated during inflammation and have been shown to be responsible for the pathological symptoms associated with allergic diseases.

In addition, PGD2 has been implicated in the regulation of sleep [25], sensation of pain [26], and the development of male reproductive organs [27].

Two isoforms of PGDS exist in humans. The hemopoetic type, H-PGDS, requires glutathione for catalysis and is primarily found in the cytoplasm [28], whereas the lipocalin type, L-PGDS, does not require glutathione for catalysis and is found in the brain, heart, and testis [29]. It is of particular interest to emphasize that among all the enzymes involved in the metabolism of prostanoids, L-PGDS is the only enzyme that has a lipocalin fold. As a lipocalin, L-PGDS has been shown to bind numerous ligands, such as retinoic acid [30], bile pigments [31], amyloid peptides [32], and gangliosides [33], and has been postulated to assist their transport.

In humans, serum L-PGDS levels have been positively associated with the severity of coronary artery disease [34], whereas in mice ablation of L-PGDS has been reported to aggravate the development of atherosclerosis [35].

However, its involvement in insulin sensitivity and glucose tolerance is less clear [36, 37]. Furthermore, in humans, *L-PGDS* expression is higher in subcutaneous adipose tissue than abdominal adipose tissue [38], suggesting it may modulate depot-specific differences in adipose tissue function.

Retinol Binding

Retinol and its derived form which are essential for vision for skin health and bone growth, because of their hydrophobic structure must be bound by specific proteins in body fluids and within cells. Plasma retinol-binding protein (RBP) and epididymal retinoic acid binding protein (ERABP) carry retinoids in body fluids, while cellular RBPs (CRBPs) and cellular retinoic acid-binding proteins (CRABPs) carry retinoids within cells [38]. All these transport proteins belong to the lipocalin family.

RBP and ERABP belong to the RBP family. CRBPs and CRABPs belong to the fatty acid-binding protein-like (FABP) family.

RBP specifically bounds retinol, delivering it from the liver stores through the blood circulation to peripheral tissues. In plasma, the RBP-retinol complex interacts with transthyretin, which prevents it from being filtered out of the blood by the kidney glomeruli. ERABP in the lumen of the epididymis is required for sperm maturation and binds both all-trans retinoic acid and 9-cis retinoic acid. There are four different CRBPs lipocalins: CRBP I, II, III, and IV. They are highly homologous proteins but have distinct tissue distributions and retinoid-binding properties. Among these CRBPs, mammalian CRBP I and II are the best-characterized members of the CRBP family and are known to bind all-trans retinol and all-trans retinal with a high affinity but not all-trans retinoic acid [38-42]. CRABPs may regulate the interactions between retinoic acids and their nuclear receptors by regulating the concentration of retinoic acids present [43-45].

Conclusion

The lipocalin family exhibits a variety of physiological roles. The proteins in the lipocalin family are involved in immune and inflammatory response and cellular detoxification. They work as mammalian lipocalin allergens with their poor capacity to stimulate the cellular immune system. They are also involved in the transport of mammalian pheromones, PG synthesis, and retinol binding.

References

[1]   Fournier, T., Medjoubi-N N., Porquet, D. Alpha-1-acid glycoprotein. *Biochim. Biophys. Acta* 2000;1482:157-71.

[2]   Akerstrom, B., Logdberg, L., Berggard, T., Osmark, P., Lindqvist, A. alpha (1)-Microglobulin: a yellow-brown lipocalin. *Biochim. Biophys. Acta* 2000;1482:172-84.

[3]   Zhang, Y., Gao, Z., Guo, Z., Zhang, H., Zhang, Z., Luo, M., Hou, H., Huang, A., Dong, Y., Wang, D. The crystal structure of human protein α1M reveals a chromophore-binding site and two putative protein-protein interfaces. *Biochem. Biophys. Res. Commun.* 2013;439:346-50.

[4]   Seppälä, M., Taylor, R. N., Koistinen, H., Koistinen, R., Milgrom, E. Glycodelin: a major lipocalin protein of the reproductive axis with diverse actions in cell recognition and differentiation. *Endocr. Rev.* 2002;23:401-30.

[5]   Kjcldsen, L., Cowland, J. B., Borregaard, N. Human neutrophil gelatinase-associated lipocalin and homologous proteins in rat and mouse. *Biochim. Biophys. Acta* 2000;1482:272-83.

[6]   Schreck, S. F., Parker, C., Plumb, M. E., Sodetz, J. M. Human complement protein C8Q. *Biochim. Biophys. Acta* 2000;1482:199-208.

[7]   Kasper, S., Matusik, R. J. Rat probasin: structure and function of an outlier lipocalin. *Biochim. Biophys. Acta* 2000;1482:249-58.

[8]   Urade, Y., Hayaishi, O. Biochemical, structural, genetic, physiological, and pathophysiological features of lipocalin type prostaglandin D synthase. *Biochim. Biophys. Acta* 2000;1482:259-71.

[9]   Goetz, D. H., Holmes, M. A., Borregaard, N., Bluhm, M. E., Raymond, K. N., Strong, R. K. The neutrophil lipocalin NGAL is a bacteriostatic agent that interferes with siderophore-mediated iron acquisition. *Mol. Cell* 2002;10:1033–43.

[10]   Fischbach, M. A., Lin, H., Zhou, L., Yu, Y., Aberge, R. J., Liu, D. R., Raymond, K. N., Wanner, B. I., Strong, R. K., Walsh, C. T., Aderem, A., Smith, K. D. The pathogen-associated iroA gene cluster mediates bacterial evasion of lipocalin 2. *PNAS* 2006;103:16502–07.

[11]   Smith, K. D. Iron metabolism at the host pathogen interface: Lipocalin 2 and the pathogen-associated *iron* gene cluster. *Int. J. Biochem. Cell Biol.* 2007;39:1776–80.

[12]   Mori, K., Lee, H. T., Rapoport, D., Drexler, I. R., Foster, K., Yang, J., Schmidt-Ott, K. M., Chen, X., Li, J. Y., Weiss, S., Mishra, J., Cheema, F. H., Markowitz, G., Suganami, T., Sawai, K., Mukoyama, M., Kunis, C., D'Agati, V., Devarajan, P., Barasch, J. Endocytic delivery of lipocalin-siderophore iron complex rescues the kidney from ischemia-reperfusin injury. *J. Clin. Invest.* 2005;115:610–21.

[13]   Fluckinger, M., Haas, H., Merschak, P., Glasgow, B. J., Redl, B. Human tear lipocalin exhibits antimicrobial activity by scavenging microbial siderophores. *Antimicrob. Agents Chemother.* 2004;48:3367–72.

[14] Charron, J. B., Ouellet, F., Houde, M., Sarhan, F. The plant apolipo-protein D ortholog protects *Arabidopsis* against oxidative stress. *BMC Plant Biol.* 2008;8:86.

[15] Ganfornina, M. D., Do Carmo, S., Lora, J. M., Torres-Schumann, S., Vogel, M., Allhorn, M., González, C., Bastiani, M. J., Rassart, E., Sanchez, D. Apolipoprotein D is involved in the mechanisms regulating protection from oxidative stress. *Aging Cell* 2008;7:506–15.

[16] Virtanen, T., Kinnunen, T., Rytkönen-Nissinen, M. Mammalian lipoca-lin allergens--insights into their enigmatic allergenicity. *Clin. Exp. Allergy* 2012;42:494-504.

[17] Parviainen, S., Kinnunen, T., Rytkönen-Nissinen, M., Nieminen, A., Liukko, A., Virtanen, T. Mammal-derived respiratory lipocalin allergens do not exhibit dendritic cell-activating capacity. *Scand. J. Immunol.* 2013;77:171–6.

[18] Stopková, R., Hladovcová, D., Kokavec, J., Vyoral, D., Stopka, P. Multiple roles of secretary lipocalins (Mup, Obp) in mice. *Folia Zool.* 2009;58:29–40.

[19] Lacazette, E., Gachon, A. M., Pitiot, G. A novel human odorant-binding protein gene family resulting from genomic duplicons at 9q34: differen-tial expression in the oral and genital sphere. *Human Mol. Genet.* 2000; 9:289–301.

[20] Dear, T. N., Campbell, K., Rabbitts, T. H. Molecular cloning of putative odorant-binding and odorant metabolizing proteins. *Biochemistry* 1991; 30:10376–82.

[21] Pevsner, J., Hou, V., Snowman, A. M., Snyder, S. H. Odorant-binding Protein, Characterization of ligand binding. *J. Biol. Chem.* 1990:265: 6118–25.

[22] Taylor, A. J., Cook, D. J., Scott, D. J. Role of odorant binding proteins: Comparing hypothetical mechanisms with experimental data. *Chem. Percept.* 2008;1:153–62.

[23] Clausen, J. Proteins in normal cerebrospinal fluid not found in serum. *Proc. Soc. Exp. Biol. Med.* 1961;107:170-72.

[24] Nagata, A., Suzuki, Y., Igarashi, M., Eguchi, N., Toh, H., Urade, Y., Hayaishi, O. Human brain prostaglandin D synthase has been evolution-arily differentiated from lipophilic-ligand carrier proteins. *Proc. Natl. Acad. Sci. US 1*991;88:4020-4.

[25] Hoffmann, A., Conradt, H. S., Gross, G., Nimtz, M., Lottspeich, F., Wurster, U. Purification and chemical characterization of beta-trace

protein from human cerebrospinal fluid: its identification as prostaglandin-D synthase. *J. Neurochem.* 1993;61:451–56.

[26] Qu, W. M., Huang, Z. L., Xu, X. H., Aritake, K., Eguchi, N., Nambu, F., Narumiya, S., Urade, Y., Hayaishi, O. Lipocalin-type prostaglandin D synthase produces prostaglandin D2 involved in regulation of physiological sleep. *Proc. Natl. Acad. Sci. US* 2006;103:17949–54.

[27] Eguchi, N., Minami, T., Shirafuji, N., Kanaoka, Y., Tanaka, T., Nagata, A., Yoshida, N., Urade, Y., Ito, S., Hayaishi, O. Lack of tactile pain (allodynia) in lipocalin-type prostaglandin D synthase-deficient mice. *Proc. Natl. Acad. Sci. US* 1999;96:726–30.

[28] Malki, S., Nef, S., Notarnicola, C., Thevenet, L., Gasca, P., Mejean, C., Berta, P., Poulat, F., Boizet-Bonhoure, B. Prostaglandin D2 induces nuclear import of the sex-determining factor SOX9 via its cAMP-PKA phosphorylation. *EMBO J.* 2005;24:1798–1809.

[29] Kanaoka, Y., Ago, H., Inagaki, E., Nanayama, T., Miyano, M., Kikuno, R., Fujii, Y., Eguchi, N., Toh, H., Urade, Y., Hayaishi, O. Cloning and crystal structure of hematopoietic prostaglandin D synthase. *Cell* 1997; 90:1085–95.

[30] Urade, Y., Hayaishi, O. Biochemical, structural, genetic, physiological, and pathophysiological features of lipocalin- type prostaglandin D synthase. *Biochim. Biophys. Acta* 2000;1482:259–71.

[31] Tanaka, T., Urade, Y., Kimura, H., Eguchi, N., Nishikawa, A., Hayaishi, O. Lipocalin-type prostaglandin D synthase (-trace) is a newly recognized type of retinoid transporter. *J. Biol. Chem.* 1997;272:15789–95.

[32] Beuckmann, C. T., Aoyagi, M., Okazaki, I., Hiroike, T., Toh, H., Hayaishi, O., Urade, Y. Binding of biliverdin, bilirubin, and thyroid hormones to lipocalin-type prostaglandin D synthase. *Biochemistry* 1999;38:8006–13.

[33] Hansson, S. F., Andreasson, U., Wall, M., Skoog, I., Andreasen, N., Wallin, A., Zetterberg, H., Blennow, K. Reduced levels of amyloid-beta-binding proteins in cerebrospinal fluid from Alzheimer's disease patients. *J. Alzheimers Dis.* 2009;16:389–97.

[34] Mohri, I., Taniike, M., Okazaki, I., Kagitani-Shimono, K., Aritake, K., Kanekiyo, T., Yagi, T., Takikita, S., Kim, H. S., Urade, Y., Suzuki, K. Lipocalin-type prostaglandin D synthase is up-regulated in oligodendrocytes in lysosomal storage diseases and binds gangliosides. *J. Neurochem.* 2006;97:641–51.

[35] Inoue, T., Eguchi, Y., Matsumoto, T., Kijima, Y., Kato, Y., Ozaki, Y., Waseda, K., Oda, H., Seiki, K., Node, K., Urade, Y. Lipocalin-type prostaglandin D synthase is a powerful biomarker for severity of stable coronary artery disease. *Atherosclerosis* 2008;201:385–91.

[36] Tanaka, R., Miwa, Y., Mou, K., Tomikawa, M., Eguchi, N., Urade, Y., Takahashi-Yanaga, F., Morimoto, S., Wake, N., Sasaguri, T. Knockout of the l-pgds gene aggravates obesity and atherosclerosis in mice. *Biochem. Biophys. Res. Commun.* 2009;378:851–56.

[37] Ragolia, L., Palaia, T., Hall, C. E., Maesaka, J. K., Eguchi, N., Urade, Y. Accelerated glucose intolerance, nephropathy and atherosclerosis in prostaglandin D2 synthase knockout mice. *J. Biol. Chem.* 2005;280: 29946-55.

[38] Quinkler, M., Bujalska, I. J., Tomlinson, J. W., Smith, D. M., Stewart, P. M. Depot-specific prostaglandin synthesis in human adipose tissue: a novel possible mechanism of adipogenesis. *Gene* 2006;380:137–43.

[39] Folli, C., Calderone, V., Ottonello, S., Bolchi, A., Zanotti, G., Stoppini, M., Berni, R. Identification, retinoid binding, and x-ray analysis of a human retinol-binding protein. *Proc. Natl. Acad. Sci. US* 2001;98:3710–15.

[40] Marcelino, A. M., Smock, R. G., Gierasch, L. M. Evolutionary coupling of structural and functional sequence information in the intracellular lipid-binding protein family. *Proteins* 2006;63:373–84.

[41] Lu, J., Cistola, D. P., Li, E. Two homologous rat cellular retinol-binding proteins differ in local conformational flexibility. *J. Mol. Biol.* 2003; 330:799–812.

[42] Franzoni, L., Lucke, C., Perez, C., Cavazzini, D., Rademacher, M., Ludwig, C., Spisni, A., Rossi, G. L., Rüterjans, H. Structure and backbone dynamics of Apo- and holo-cellular retinol-binding protein in solution. *J. Biol. Chem.* 2002;277:21983–97.

[43] Folli, C., Calderone, V., Ramazzina, I., Zanotti, G., Berni, R. Ligand binding and structural analysis of a human putative cellular retinol-binding protein. *J. Biol. Chem.* 2002;277:41970-77.

[44] Donovan, M., Olofsson, B., Gustafson, A. L., Dencker, L., Eriksson, U. The cellular retinoic acid binding proteins. *J. Steroid Biochem. Mol. Biol.* 1995;53:459–65.

[45] Kleywegt, G. J., Bergfors, T., Senn, H., Le Motte, P., Gsell, B., Shudo, K., Jones, T. A. Crystal structures of cellular retinoic acid binding proteins I and II in complex with all trans-retinoic acid and a synthetic retinoid. *Structure* 1994;2:1241–58.

In: Neutrophil Gelatinase-Associated Lipocalin   ISBN: 978-1-63117-984-6
Editors: M. Hur and S. Di Somma   © 2014 Nova Science Publishers, Inc.

Chapter 5

Lipocalin: Cell Regulation, Cancer Cell Interaction

*Patrizia Cardelli**

Department of Molecular and Clinical Medicine, Sant'Andrea
Hospital, Sapienza University, School of Medicine, Rome, Italy

Abstract

Lipocalins are physiologically expressed in normal tissues, and some of them play an important role in cell proliferation as well as in cell differentiation. The pathways by which lipocalins regulate cell homeostasis are of both biochemical and clinical interests, because several lipocalins have an anomalous expression during the development and progression of both benign and malignant diseases.

Introduction

Lipocalins mediate cell regulation; by delivering their lipophilic ligands to target cells, by protease inhibitory activity, by immunosuppressive properties, by the binding to specific receptors and subsequent receptor - mediated intra-

---

* Corresponding author: Patrizia Cardelli. E-mail: patrizia.cardelli@uniroma1.it.

cellular signalling. However, each one of these physiological pathways can assume a particular role in cell dysregulation during cancer development.

Cellular retinol-binding protein I functions in retinol storage and its expression is lower in human cancer cells than in normal cells. In MTSV1-7 an SV40-immortalized human mammary epithelial cell line CRBP-I is down-regulated compromising retinoic acid receptor (RAR) activity, leading to loss of cell differentiation and tumor progression [1].

The same behavior was observed in serum of ovarian cancer patient where retinol binding protein-4 levels were decreased [2].

Decreased serum glycodelin concentration is related to tumor aggressiveness and poor clinical outcome in advanced ovarian cancer. Glycodelin might be an interesting marker to discriminate between high risk and low risk patients in stage III and IV ovarian cancer [3]. Another lipocalin ApoD is a marker for steroid signalling in breast cancer [4, 5], and its high affinity to arachidonic acid [6], progesterone, and tamoxifen [7] makes it a very interesting putative prognostic and predictive marker in breast cancer.

NGAL in Tumor Progression

NGAL, beside its role in many "non neoplastic" diseases, is involved in the physiopathology of tumor progression. NGAL is expressed in tumors from several organs, including thyroid [8], breast [9], lung [10], esophagus [11], ovary [12], endometrium [13], colon [14], liver, bile ducts [15], stomach [16], pancreas [17, 18], and skin [19]. NGAL expression was significantly upregulated; in ovarian tumors [20]; in endometrial hyperplasia and endometrial carcinoma [13]; in gastrointestinal tumors like colorectal, pancreatic, hepatocellular, and gastric cancers [14, 15, 17, 18]; and in hematologic malignancies including chronic myeloid leukemia, polycythemia vera, and essential thrombocythemia [21, 22].

Recently, NGAL has been proposed as a prognostic marker in colorectal cancer (CRC) where high plasma NGAL levels are associated with higher neoplastic tissue volume, characteristics of neoplastic invasion and recurrence, showing a prognostic utility mainly in metastatic CRC patients [23].

The levels of NGAL/MMP-9 complex were significantly higher in the urine and cerebrospinal fluid of patients with primitive brain tumors and returned to normal after surgical excision of the neoplastic tissue.

A relevant increase of the NGAL/MMP-9 complex was observed in oesophageal squamous cell carcinoma [11].

On gastric carcinoma tissue, Kubben et al. [24] showed that high expression of NGAL/MMP-9 correlated with the grade of malignancy.

In a murine implanted breast cancer cell line, the high expression of NGAL/MMP-9 correlated with the formation of an aggressive tumoral phenotype, with high angiogenic potential and proliferative activity [25].

Furthermore, in patients with breast tumors, NGAL/MMP-9 complexes were present in almost all of the urine samples [25].

An analysis using zimographic techniques [26] showed that there was a significant association between the expression of this complex and the aggressiveness of the tumor invasion, confirming, *in vivo,* that the association of NGAL with MMP-9 is one of the principal mechanisms underlying the tumor development induced by the protein [25].

Moreover, using a p53-null anaplastic thyroid carcinoma cell line (FRO), NGAL was found upregulated by NF-kB protein complex so an improper regulation of NF-κB could enhance cancer development [27, 28]. In apparent conflict with most of the literature, some studies have hypothesized that NGAL could inhibit the pro-neoplastic factor HIF-1α, which plays an essential role in cellular and systemic responses to hypoxia [28], FA-kinase phosphorylation, and also VEGF synthesis, suggesting that, in alternative cellular/tissue microenvironment, paradoxically, NGAL can assume anti-tumoral and anti-metastatic effect in neoplasia [29-32].

Conclusion

All the data already available need to be confirmed with further controlled studies focused on the potential use of some lipocalins, may be in a multi-markers approach, for the diagnosis, follow-up, and prognosis of tumors as well as in predicting response to the more appropriate pharmacological therapies.

References

[1]   Farias, E. F., Ong, D. E., Ghyselinck, N. B., Nakajo, S., Kuppumbatti, Y. S., Mira y Lopez, R. Cellular retinol-binding protein I, a regulator of breast epithelial retinoic acid receptor activity, cell differentiation, and tumorigenicity. *J. Natl. Cancer Inst.* 2005;97:21-9.

[2] Lorkova, L., Pospisilova, J., Lacheta, J., Leahomschi, S., Zivny, J., Cibula, D., Zivny, J., Petrak, J. Decreased concentrations of retinol-binding protein 4 in sera of epithelial ovarian cancer patients: A potential biomarker identified by proteomics. *Oncol. Rep.* 2012;27:318-24.

[3] Scholz, C., Heublein, S., Lenhard, M., Friese, K., Mayr, D., Jeschke, U. Glycodelin A is a prognostic marker to predict poor outcome in advanced stage ovarian cancer patients. *BMC Res. Notes* 2012;5:551.

[4] Søiland, H., Søreide, K., Janssen, E. A., Kørner, H., Baak, J. P., and Søreide, J. A. Emerging concepts of apolipoprotein D with possible implications for breast cancer. *Cell. Oncol.* 2007;29:195-209.

[5] Simard, J., Dauvois, S., Haagensen, D. E., Levesque, C., Merand, Y., Labrie, F. Regulation of progesterone-binding breast cyst protein GCDFP-24 secretion by estrogens and androgens in human breast cancer cells: a new marker of steroid action in breast cancer. *Endocrinology* 1990;126: 3223-31.

[6] Morais Cabral, J. H., Atkins, G. L., Sanchez, L. M., Lopez-Boado, Y. S., Lopez-Otin, C., Sawyer, L. Arachidonic acid binds to apolipoprotein D: implications for the protein's function. *FEBS Lett.* 1995;366: 53-6.

[7] Lea, O. A. Binding properties of progesterone-binding Cyst protein, PBCP. *Steroids* 1988;52:337-8.

[8] Volpe, V., Raia, Z., Sanguigno, L., Somma, D., Mastrovito, P., Moscato, F., Mellone, S., Leonardi, A., Pacifico, F. NGAL controls the metastatic potential of anaplastic thyroid carcinoma cells. *J. Clin. Endocrinol. Metab.* 2013;98:228-35.

[9] Bauer, M., Eickhoff, J. C., Gould, M. N., Mundhenke, C., Maass, N., Friedl, A. Neutrophil gelatinase-associated lipocalin (NGAL) is a pre-dictor of poor prognosis in human primary breast cancer. *Breast Cancer Res. Treat.* 2008;108:389–97.

[10] Linnerth, N. M., Sirbovan, K., Moorehead, R. A. Use of a transgenic mouse model to identify markers of human lung tumors. *Int. J. Cancer* 2005;114:977–82.

[11] Zhang, H., Xu, L., Xiao, D., Xie, J., Zeng, H., Wang, Z., Zhang, X., Niu, Y., Shen, Z., Shen, J., Wu, X., Li, E. Upregulation of neutrophil gelati-nase-associated lipocalin in oesophageal squamous cell carcinoma: significant correlation with cell differentiation and tumour invasion. *J. Clin. Pathol.* 2007;60: 555–61.

[12] Cho, H., Kim, J. H. Lipocalin2 expressions correlate significantly with tumor differentiation in epithelial ovarian cancer. *J. Histochem. Cyto-chem.* 2009;57:513–21.

[13] Miyamoto, T., Kashima, H., Suzuki, A., Kikuchi, N., Konishi, I., Seki, N., Shiozawa, T. Laser-captured microdissection-microarray analysis of the genes involved in endometrial carcinogenesis: stepwise up-regulation of lipocalin2 expression in normal and neoplastic endometria and its functional relevance. *Hum. Pathol.* 2011;42:1265–74.

[14] Bousserouel, S., Kauntz, H., Gosse, F., Bouhadjar, M., Soler, L., Marescaux, J., Raul, F. Identification of gene expression profiles correlated to tumor progression in a preclinical model of colon carcinogenesis. *Int. J. Oncol.* 2010;36:1485–90.

[15] Friedl, A., Stoesz, S. P., Buckley, P., Gould, M. N. Neutrophil gelatinase-associated lipocalin in normal and neoplastic human tissues. Cell type-specific pattern of expression. *Histochem. J.* 1999;31:433–41.

[16] Wang, H. J., He, X. J., Ma, Y. Y., Jiang, X. T., Xia, Y. J., Ye, Z. Y., Zhao, Z. S., Tao, H. Q. Expressions of neutrophil gelatinase-associated lipocalin in gastric cancer: a potential biomarker for prognosis and an ancillary diagnostic test. *Anat. Rec.* (Hoboken) 2010;293:1855-63.

[17] Furutani, M., Arii, S., Mizumoto, M., Kato, M., Imamura, M. Identification of a neutrophil gelatinase-associated lipocalin mRNA in human pancreatic cancers using a modified signal sequence trap method. *Cancer Lett.* 1998;122:209–14.

[18] Laurell, H., Bouisson, M., Berthelemy, P., Rochaix, P., Dejean, S., Besse, P., Susini, C., Pradayrol, L., Vaysse, N., Buscail, L. Identification of biomarkers of human pancreatic adenocarcinomas by expression profiling and validation with gene expression analysis in endoscopic ultrasound-guided fine needle aspiration samples. *World J. Gastroenterol.* 2006;12:3344–51.

[19] Mallbris, L., O'Brien, K. P., Hulthen, A., Sandstedt, B., Cowland, J. B., Borregaard, N., Stahle-Backdahl, M. Neutrophil gelatinase-associated lipocalin is a marker for dysregulated keratinocyte differentiation in human skin. *Exp. Dermatol.* 2002;11:584–91.

[20] Lim, R., Ahmed, N., Borregaard, N., Riley, C., Wafai, R., Thompson, E. W., Quinn, M. A., Rice, G. E. Neutrophil gelatinase-associated lipocalin (NGAL) an early-screening biomarker for ovarian cancer: NGAL is associated with epidermal growth factor-induced epithelio-mesenchymal transition. *Int. J. Cancer* 2007;120:2426–34.

[21] Villalva, C., Sorel, N., Bonnet, M. L., Guilhot, J., Mayeur-Rousse, C., Guilhot, F., Chomel, J. C., Turhan, A. G. Neutrophil gelatinase-associated lipocalin expression in chronic myeloid leukemia. *Leuk. Lymphoma* 2008;49:984–8.

[22] Allegra, A., Alonci, A., Bellomo, G., Campo, S., Cannavo, A., Penna, G., Russo, S., Centorrino, R., Gerace, D., Petrungaro, A., Musolino, C. Increased serum levels of neutrophil gelatinase-associated lipocalin in patients with essential thrombocythemia and polycythemia vera. *Leuk. Lymphoma* 2011;52:101–7.

[23] Martí, J., Fuster, J., Solà, A. M., Hotter, G., Molina, R., Pelegrina, A., Ferrer, J., Deulofeu, R., Fondevila, C., García-Valdecasas, J. C. Prognostic value of serum neutrophil gelatinase-associated lipocalin in metastatic and nonmetastatic colorectal cancer. *World J. Surg.* 2013;37: 1103-9.

[24] Kubben, F. J., Sier, C. F., Hawinkels, L. J., Tschesche, H., van Duijn, W., Zuidwijk, K., van der Reijden, J. J., Hanemaaijer, R., Griffioen, G., Lamers, C. B., Verspaget, H. W. Clinical evidence for a protective role of lipocalin-2 against MMP-9 autodegradation and the impact for gastric cancer. *Eur. J. Cancer* 2007;43:1869–76.

[25] Fernández, C. A., Yan, L., Louis, G., Yang, J., Kutok, J. L., Moses, M. A. The matrix metalloproteinase-9/neutrophil gelatinase-associated lipocalin complex plays a role in breast tumor growth and is present in the urine of breast cancer patients. *Clin. Cancer Res.* 2005;11:5390–5.

[26] Yan, L., Borregaard, N., Kjeldsen, L., Moses, M. A. The high molecular weight urinary matrix metalloproteinase (MMP) activity is a complex of gelatinase B/MMP-9 and neutrophil gelatinase-associated lipocalin (NGAL): modulation of MMP-9 activity by NGAL. *J. Biol. Chem.* 2001; 276: 37258–65.

[27] Iannetti, A., Pacifico, F., Acquaviva, R., Lavorgna, A., Crescenzi, E., Vascotto, C., Tell, G., Salzano, A. M., Scaloni, A., Vuttariello, E., Chiappetta, G., Formisano, S., Leonardi, A. The neutrophil gelatinase-associated lipocalin (NGAL), a NF-kappaB-regulated gene, is a survival factor for thyroid neoplastic cells. *Proc. Nat. Acad. Sci. US* 2008;105: 14058–63.

[28] Rius, J., Guma, M., Schachtrup, C., Akassoglou, K., Zinkernagel, A. S., Nizet, V., Johnson, R. S., Haddad, G. G., Karin, M. NF-kappaB links innate immunity to the hypoxic response through transcriptional regulation of HIF-1alpha. *Nature* 2008;453: 807–11.

[29] Hanai, J., Mammoto, T., Seth, P., Mori, K., Karumanchi, S. A., Barasch, J., Sukhatme, V. P. Lipocalin 2 diminishes invasiveness and metastasis of Ras-transformed cells. *J. Biol. Chem.* 2005;280:3641–7.

[30] Venkatesha, S., Hanai, J., Seth, P., Karumanchi, S. A., Sukhatme, V. P. Lipocalin 2 antagonizes the proangiogenic action of ras in transformed cells. *Mol. Cancer Res.* 2006;4:821–9.

[31] Tong, Z., Kunnumakkara, A. B., Wang, H., Matsuo, Y., Diagaradjane, P., Harikumar, K. B., Ramachandran, V., Sung, B., Chakraborty, A., Bresalier, R. S., Logsdon, C., Aggarwal, B. B., Krishnan, S., Guha, S. Neutrophil gelatinase-associated lipocalin: a novel suppressor of invasion and angiogenesis in pancreatic cancer. *Cancer Res.* 2008;68: 6100–8.

[32] Lee, H. J., Lee, E. K., Lee, K. J., Hong, S. W., Yoon, Y., Kim, J. S. Ectopic expression of neutrophil gelatinase-associated lipocalin suppresses the invasion and liver metastasis of colon cancer cells. *Int. J. Cancer* 2006;118:2490–7.

In: Neutrophil Gelatinase-Associated Lipocalin   ISBN: 978-1-63117-984-6
Editors: M. Hur and S. Di Somma   © 2014 Nova Science Publishers, Inc.

Chapter 6

Urinary versus Plasma NGAL

Giorgio Zampini, Benedetta De Berardinis
and Salvatore Di Somma[*]
Department of Emergency Medicine, Department of Medical-Surgery
Sciences and Translational Medicine, University Sapienza Rome,
Sant'Andrea Hospital, Italy

Abstract

In the currently available literature there are only few studies which accurately evaluated and/or compared the analytical characteristics and performance of NGAL assay methods. Furthermore, the majority of the clinical studies report insufficient data on the analytical performance of the method used for NGAL assay. Recently certified assays for the clinical chemistry platform, using either plasma or urine samples for measurement of NGAL, have been introduced, although the number of studies using these methods is still small. The results of a recent meta-analysis indicate that the serum/plasma and urine samples have similar diagnostic accuracies in predicting the presence of AKI.

[*] Correspondence: salvatore.disomma@uniroma1.it.

Introduction

The first analytical procedure set up for the measurement of NGAL in blood or urine samples were based on ELISA [1, 2] or immunoblotting systems [3]. In general, these methods are manual, not standardized methods, which are not recommended for clinical routine tests, but only for research studies [1 - 7]. The measurement of NGAL in serum, plasma, and urine samples can be also performed by means of a commercially available ELISA kit (NGAL Rapid ELISA KIT 037, Antibodyshop ELISA kit, BioPorto Diagnostics, Denmark) using both a manual procedure [4, 6] or several chemistry analyzers [7]. The analytical performance of this ELISA kit was evaluated by Pedersen et al. [6] using the manual procedure for the measurement of NGAL in both urine and plasma samples.

A point-of-care test (POCT) method (Triage Biosite, Alere Healthcare) is a commercial fluorescence-based immunoassay for a rapid measurement (approximately 30 min) of NGAL in EDTA anti-coagulated whole blood or plasma samples [8 - 10]. This POCT method has a lower detection limit at 15 ng/mL and the upper limit of the measurable range at 1,300 ng/mL [8, 10]. More recently, a chemiluminescent microparticle immunoassay (CMIA) method became commercially available; using the automated platform ARCHITECT (Abbott Diagnostics) for the measurement of NGAL both in blood and urine samples [9 - 11]. This assay involves a micro-particle reagent prepared by covalently attaching an anti-NGAL antibody to paramagnetic particles and a conjugate reagent prepared by labeling a second anti-NGAL antibody with acridinium. The analytical characteristics of this CMIA method have been evaluated by Grenier et al. [11]. In particular, this method showed a close linear regression with an ELISA kit (AntibodyShop NGAL Rapid ELISA Kit, BioPorto, Denmark) throughout all NGAL concentration interval tested, ranging from 2 to 1,500 µg/L (R = 0.994, n = 100; ARCHITECT = 0.93 ELISA + 4.2) [11]. Moreover, the imprecision at the lower limit of measurable range (i.e., 2 µg/L) was < 20% [11].

Reference Values

There are no studies intentionally set up with the aim to accurately evaluate the reference values of NGAL measurement in blood or urine specimens using large reference populations, stratified according to age, gender, and ethnicity. However, some authors reported "normal values" measured in relatively large groups, including apparently healthy subjects, enrolled in a clinical study as a control group. Furthermore, some information on the "expected normal values" is usually reported in the product inserts of the commercial NGAL assays, distributed by the manufacturers. The expected range of NGAL normal values of Triage NGAL Test, as reported by the manufacturer, was 149 ng/mL with a 90 % confidence interval ranging from 100 to 194 ng/mL [10]. The kit insert of the CMIA assay, distributed by Abbott Diagnostics [12], reports a value of 132 µg/L as the 95th percentile of NGAL values. However, reference ranges, adjusted for age, gender, and ethnicity, as well as reliable cutoff values, calculated on large patient population, for ruling in and out of acute kidney injury (AKI) syndromes, are still lacking.

Blood versus Urine

By now there is no common consensus on the type of sample (blood or urine) more appropriate to perform the dosage. It is believed that plasma levels of NGAL may be influenced by extra renal factors, while an increase of the marker in the urine provide a more specific estimation of renal tubular damage. On the other hand, the collection of blood, although invasive, is generally less complex than urine collection; and in most cases, blood collection is performed for testing the other laboratory parameters except for NGAL, so the same sample can be used for NGAL measurement. Urine samples are certainly preferred in infants. However, the urinary sampling is very difficult in incontinent patients, requiring bladder catheterization, and it is impossible in anuric patients.

Conclusion

In the emergency setting, the use of a rapid POCT system provides quantitative NGAL results from whole blood in 15 minutes. It adds important clinical implications since the time to diagnosis in this emergency setting is inversely related to the optimal patient outcome. Inherent to this is prompt initiation of treatment and timely patient disposition [13]. The results of a recent meta-analysis indicate that the serum/plasma and urine samples have similar diagnostic accuracies in predicting the presence of AKI [14].

References

[1]   Mishra J, Dent C, Tarabishi R, Mitsnefes MM, Ma Q, Kelly C, Ruff SM, Zahedi K, Shao M, Bean J, Mori K, Barasch J, Devarajan P. Neutrophil gelatinase-associated lipocalin (NGAL) as a biomarker for acute renal injury after cardiac surgery. *Lancet* 2005;365:1231–8.

[2]   Stejskal D, Karpísek M, Humenanska V, Hanulova Z, Stejskal P, Kusnierova P, Petzel M. Lipocalin-2: development, analytical characterization, and clinical testing of a new ELISA. *Horm Metab Res* 2008;40:381-5.

[3]   Wagener G, Jan M, Kim M, Mori K, Barasch JM, Sladen RN, Lee HT. Association between increases in urinary neutrophil gelatinase associated lipocalin and acute renal dysfunction after adult cardiac surgery. *Anesthesiology* 2006;105:485–91.

[4]   Bachorzewska-Gajewska H, Malyszko J, Sitniewska E, Malyszko JS, Dobrzycki S. Neutrophil-gelatinase-associated lipocalin and renal function after percutaneous coronary interventions. Am J Nephrol 2006;26:287–92.

[5]   Cai L, Borowiec J, Xu S, Han W, Venge P. Assays of urine levels of HNL/NGAL in patients undergoing cardiac surgery and the impact of antibody configuration on their clinical performances. *Clin Chim Acta* 2009;403:121–5.

[6]   Pedersen KR, Ravn HB, Hjortdal VE, N ø rregaard R, Povlsen JV. Neutrophil gelatinase-associated lipocalin (NGAL): validation of commercially available ELISA. *Scand J Clin Lab Invest* 2010;70:374–82.

[7]   NGAL Rapid ELISA kit (KIT 037). Information included in the commercial web site (*http://www.ngal.com/*).

[8]   Heyne N, Kemmner S, Schneider C, Nadalin S, Königsrainer A, Häring HU. Urinary neutrophil gelatinase-associated lipocalin accurately detects acute allograft rejection among other causes of acute kidney injury in renal allograft recipients. *Transplantation* 2012;93:1252-7.

[9]   Ronco C, Cruz D, Noland BW. Neutrophil gelatinase-associated lipocalin curve and neutrophil gelatinase-associated lipocalin extended-

range assay: a new biomarker approach in the early diagnosis of acute kidney injury and cardio-renal syndrome. *Semin Nephrol* 2012;32:121-8.

[10] Triage NGAL Test. Biosite, *Product insert*. Inverness Medical, 1000378 v1 01/12, 01/03/2012.

[11] Grenier FC, Ali S, Syed H, Workman R, Martens F, Liao M, Wang Y, Wong PY. Evaluation of the ARCHITECT urine NGAL assay: assay performance, specimen handling requirements and biological variability. *Clin Biochem* 2010;43:615–20.

[12] Urine NGAL (REF 1P37). *Product insert*. Abbott Diagnostics Division, Longford, Ireland, 2009.

[13] Di Somma S, Magrini L, De Berardinis B, Marino R, Ferri E, Moscatelli P, Ballarino P, Carpinteri G, Noto P, Gliozzo B, Paladino L, Di Stasio E. Additive value of blood neutrophil gelatinase-associated lipocalin to clinical judgement in acute kidney injury diagnosis and mortality prediction in patients hospitalized from the emergency department. *Crit Care.* 2013;17:R29.

[14] Koyner J, Bennett M, Worcester E, Ma Q, Raman J, JeevanandamV, Kasza KE, O'Connor MF, Konczal DJ, Trevino S, Devarajan P, Murray PT. Urinary cystatin C as an early biomarker of acute kidney injury following adult cardiothoracic surgery. *Kidney Int* 2008;74:1059–69.

In: Neutrophil Gelatinase-Associated Lipocalin   ISBN: 978-1-63117-984-6
Editors: M. Hur and S. Di Somma   © 2014 Nova Science Publishers, Inc.

Chapter 7

History of NGAL Assays

Patrizia Cardelli[*1] *and Laura Magrini*[2]

[1]Department of Molecular and Clinical Medicine, Sant'Andrea Hospital,
Sapienza University, School of Medicine, Rome, Italy
[2]Department of Emergency Medicine, Department of Medical-Surgery
Sciences and Translational Medicine, University Sapienza Rome,
Sant'Andrea Hospital, Italy

Abstract

A brief history of the development of NGAL assays on different biological fluid from the first manual radioimmunoassay to the completely automated methods performed on point-of-care testing as well as on clinical chemistry analyzers is reported in this chapter. Some have been developed mainly for the research purposes, and the others are clinically available on automated platforms as well as on POCT instrument. Recently certified assays for clinical chemistry platform, using either plasma or urine samples for measurement of NGAL, have been introduced, although the number of studies using these methods is still small.

---

[*] correspondence: patrizia.cardelli@uniroma1.it.

Introduction

The history of the NGAL assay started at the end of the 20th century when the first data on body fluid using a radioimmunoassay became available [1]. One year later, Blaser et al. [2], using a sandwich-ELISA, determined the content of NGAL in the plasma of 122 healthy people. The plasma concentration of NGAL was log normally distributed, ranging from 25 to 211 ug/L with an average value of 97 ± 81 ug/L. The concentration of NGAL was higher when measured in serum then in plasma, even though serum and plasma values were significantly correlated. It is important to underline that this difference is due to the release of NGAL by degranulation of the neutrophils during clotting [2].

In 1996, Kjeldsen et al. [3] presented two sandwich ELISAs, one with polyclonal antibodies and the other with a mixture of polyclonal and monoclonal antibodies. The results of both assays were equally reproducible, accurate, and at least one order of magnitude better in sensitivity -detection limits of about 32 ng/L- than that obtained in the preceding years. Ten years later, in 2005, Mishra et al. [4] developed and validated an ELISA procedure for NGAL in human urine and serum using commercially available antibodies, in order to confirm and better quantify the data by an immunoblot system. The standard curves were linear between 1 − 1,000 ug/L with an intra-assay coefficient less than 5%. All these assay procedures required up to 24 hours, were manually performed, and were not standardized. They may be suitable for researches but not for clinical purpose [4 - 9].

Update in NGAL Assays

Nowadays, NGAL can be measured in serum, plasma, and urine samples using commercially available kits with different features; manual or semi-automated ELISA kit (NGAL Rapid ELISA KIT 037, Antibodyshop ELISA kit, test is a fluorescence-based immunoassay for a rapid BioPorto Diagnostics) [5, 10], immunoassays automated on several chemistry analyzers or point-of-care testing (POCT). So far, a unique POCT method (Triage, Biosite, Alere) is commercially available; it measures NGAL in EDTA anti-coagulated whole blood or plasma samples within 20 minutes [11]. The lower detection limit of this method is 15 ng/mL and the upper limit is 1,300 ng/mL [12, 13], with a proposed confidence interval between 100 - 194 ng/mL.

Actually, a particle-enhanced turbidimetric immunoassay (PETIA) for the quantitative determination of NGAL from BioPorto Diagnostics can be adapted to a variety of clinical chemistry analyzers, giving almost all laboratories immediate access to a fast and easy method to measure this analyte. This immunoassay which can be performed using EDTA plasma or urine samples is available for most popular analyzers from Abbott, Bekman, Roche, and Siemens. The assay time is approximately 10 minutes; the lower detection limit of this method is 25 ng/mL; and the upper limit is 5,000 ng/mL. The proposed reference range is 37 - 106 ng/mL in plasma and 0.7 - 9.8 ng/mL in urine samples.

More recently, a chemiluminscent microparticle immunoassay (CMIA) method for the measurement of NGAL in urine samples became commercially available, using the automated platform ARCHITECT (Abbott Diagnostics) [11, 14]. The assay time is approximately of 20 minutes; the lower detection limit is 2 ng/mL; and the upper limit is 1,500 ng/mL. Grenier et al. [14] evaluated the mean and median urine NGAL concentrations of 22.7 ng/mL (SD = 41.3 ng/mL) and 12.4 ng/mL in an apparently healthy population.

Conclusion

So far, several commercial assays have been developed for NGAL measurement. Some have been developed mainly for the research purposes, and the others are clinically available on automated platforms as well as on POCT instrument. From a practical point of view, POCT technique could be more suitable for routine and emergency NGAL measurements.

References

[1]   Xu SY, Petersson CG, Carlson M, Venge P. The development of an assay for human neutrophil lipocalin (HNL)--to be used as a specific marker of neutrophil activity in vivo and vitro. J Immunol Methods 1994;171:245-52.

[2]   Bläser J, Triebel S, Tschesche H. A sandwich enzyme immunoassay for the determination of neutrophil lipocalin in body fluids. *Clin Chim Acta* 1995;235:137-45.

[3]   Kjeldsen L, Koch C, Arnljots K, Borregaard N. Characterization of two ELISAs for NGAL, a newly described lipocalin in human neutrophils. *J Immunol Methods* 1996;198:155-64.

[4]   Mishra J, Dent C, Tarabishi R, Mitsnefes MM, Ma Q, Kelly C, Ruff SM, Zahedi K, Shao M, Bean J, Mori K, Barasch J, Devarajan P. Neutrophil gelatinase-associated lipocalin (NGAL) as a biomarker for acute renal injury after cardiac surgery. *Lancet* 2005;365:1231-8.

[5]   Bachorzewska-Gajewska H, Malyszko J, Sitniewska E, Malyszko JS, Dobrzycki S. Neutrophil-gelatinase-associated lipocalin and renal function after percutaneous coronary interventions. *Am J Nephrol* 2006;26:287–92.

[6]   Cai L, Borowiec J, Xu S, Han W, Venge P. Assays of urine levels of HNL/NGAL in patients undergoing cardiac surgery and the impact of antibody configuration on their clinical performances. *Clin Chim Acta* 2009;403:121–5.

[7]   Stejskal D, Karpísek M, Humenanska V, Hanulova Z, Stejskal P, Kusnierova P, Petzel M. Lipocalin-2: development, analytical characterization, and clinical testing of a new ELISA. *Horm Metab Res* 2008;40:381–5.

[8]   Pedersen KR, Ravn HB, Hjortdal VE, N ø rregaard R, Povlsen JV. Neutrophil gelatinase-associated lipocalin (NGAL): validation of commercially available ELISA. *Scand J Clin Lab Invest* 2010;70:374–82.

[9]   Wagener G, Jan M, Kim M, Mori K, Barasch JM, Sladen RN, Lee HT. Association between increases in urinary neutrophil gelatinase-associated lipocalin and acute renal dysfunction after adult cardiac surgery. *Anesthesiology* 2006;105:485–91.

[10] Huynh TK, Bateman DA, Parravicini E, Lorenz JM, Nemerofsky SL, Sise ME, Bowman TM, Polesana E, Barasch JM. Reference values of urinary neutrophil gelatinase-associated lipocalin in very low birth weight infants. *Pediatr Res* 2009;66:528–32.

[11] Ronco C, Cruz D, Noland BW. Neutrophil gelatinase-associated lipocalin curve and neutrophil gelatinase-associated lipocalin extended-range assay: a new biomarker approach in the early diagnosis of acute kidney injury and cardio-renal syndrome. *Semin Nephrol* 2012;32:121-8.

[12] Triage NGAL Test. *Biosite, Product insert*. Inverness Medical, 1000378 v1 01/12, 01/03/2012.

[13] Dent CL, Ma Q, Dastrala S, Bennett M, Mitsnefes MM, Barasch J, Devarajan P. Plasma neutrophil gelatinase-associated lipocalin predicts

acute kidney injury, morbidity and mortality after pediatric cardiac surgery: a prospective uncontrolled cohort study. *Crit Care* 2007;11:R127.

[14] Grenier FC, Ali S, Syed H, Workman R, Martens F, Liao M, Wang Y, Wong PY. Evaluation of the ARCHITECT urine NGAL assay: assay performance, specimen handling requirements and biological variability. *Clin Biochem* 2010;43:615–20.

In: Neutrophil Gelatinase-Associated Lipocalin   ISBN: 978-1-63117-984-6
Editors: M. Hur and S. Di Somma   © 2014 Nova Science Publishers, Inc.

Chapter 8

Diagnostic Performances of NGAL Assays

Patrizia Cardelli*¹ and Laura Magrini²

¹Department of Molecular and Clinical Medicine, Sant'Andrea Hospital,
Sapienza University School of Medicine, Rome, Italy
²Department of Emergency Medicine, Department of Medical-Surgery
Sciences and Translational Medicine, University Sapienza Rome,
Sant'Andrea Hospital, Italy

Abstract

In the currently available literature there are only few studies which accurately evaluated and/or compared the analytical characteristics and performance of NGAL assay methods. Furthermore, the majority of the clinical studies report insufficient data on the analytical performance of the method used for NGAL assay. This lack of information does not allow an accurate evaluation and/or comparison of the analytical efficacy and reliability of NGAL measurement. The few studies presented in this chapter are the representatives of growing literature in this field of interest. All the studies seem to support the finding that plasma and/or urine NGAL has a very good diagnostic performance in the early detection of AKI that is a complication of different diseases.

* Correspondence: patrizia.cardelli@uniroma1.it.

Introduction

When an emerging biomarker is proposed for clinical use, an important aspect is the characterization and validation of an assay as an early phase of the translational pathway. It is often difficult to understand and to compare data across studies and to assess the technical validity of the measurements because experimental results should be obtained by using certified assays on clinical chemistry platform or research use only (RUO) immunoassay. So far, the majority of the studies involving measurements of plasma or urinary NGAL were performed using RUO ELISAs or a certified point-of-care testing, the Triage (Alere). Recently, certified assays (BioPorto) for clinical chemistry platform, either for plasma or urine samples, have been introduced. However, the number of studies using these assays is still limited.

Performance of NGAL Assays

In a cross-sectional pilot study, Dent et al. [1] showed, using 40 plasma samples, that NGAL measurements by research ELISA and by the Triage NGAL device were highly correlated. In a subsequent study on 120 patients undergoing cardiopulmonary bypass (CPB), acute kidney injury (AKI) developed in 45 patients. The diagnosis using serum creatinine was delayed by 2 - 3 days after CPB [1], while mean plasma NGAL concentration by the Triage NGAL device increased 3-fold within 2 hours after CPB and remained significantly elevated for the duration of the study. By multivariate analysis, plasma NGAL concentration at 2 hours post-CPB time was the most powerful independent predictor of AKI. The area under the receiver operating characteristic curve (AUC) was 0.96, sensitivity was 0.84, and specificity was 0.94 for the prediction of AKI using a cut-off value of 150 µg/L. The 2-hour postoperative plasma NGAL concentrations strongly correlated with changes in creatinine concentrations, duration of AKI, and length of hospital stay. The 12-hour plasma NGAL concentration strongly correlated with mortality ($r = 0.48$, $P = 0.004$) and all measures of morbidity mentioned above [1, 2].

In a recent study on 616 patients, 21% of whom were classified as AKI, the highest median levels of plasma NGAL were in the AKI group (146 – 174 ng/mL at various time points) and increased with AKI severity (207 – 244 ng/mL for AKI Network [AKIN] classification stage > 2) [3]. The discriminative ability of plasma NGAL for AKI diagnosis (AUC, 0.77 – 0.82

at various time points) improved with higher grades of severity (AUC, 0.85 – 0.89 for AKIN > 2). Plasma NGAL discriminated AKI from normal renal function and transient azotemia (AUC, 0.85 and 0.73, respectively).

A study on 100 consecutive patients, with normal serum creatinine undergoing angiographic examinations, revealed that the serum NGAL at 2 hours (cutoff value of 106 ng/mL, sensitivity 96%, specificity 89%, and AUC 0.95), urine NGAL at 4 hours (cutoff value of 106 ng/mL, sensitivity 95%, specificity 100%, and AUC 0.96), and serum cystatin C at 24 hours after angiographic procedure can detect contrast-induced AKI earlier than serum creatinine [4].

In another study on 231 critically ill patients with suspected sepsis, the concentration of plasma NGAL was significantly different (95 [16 – 129] ng/mL; 149 [19 – 1,300] ng/mL; 245 [33 – 1,300] ng/mL; 605 [55 – 1,300] ng/mL; and 462 [127 – 1,300] ng/mL, respectively), according to the five groups of procalcitonin concentration (0.05 ng/mL, group I [healthy]; 0.05 – 0.49 ng/mL, group II [local infection]; 0.5 – 1.99 ng/mL, group III [systemic infection or sepsis]; 2.0 – 9.99 ng/mL, group IV [severe sepsis]; and $\geq$ 10 ng/mL, group V [septic shock]) ($P < 0.0001$). The concentration of plasma NGAL was also significantly different according to the renal subscore of the sepsis-related organ failure assessment (SOFA) score ($P < 0.0001$). Plasma NGAL was significantly increased in the patients with AKI compared with those without AKI (416.5 ng/mL vs. 181.0 ng/mL, $P = 0.0223$). Plasma NGAL seemed to be a highly performing predictor for AKI in patients with sepsis [5].

Recently, a urine NGAL immunoassay has been developed for a standardized clinical platform (ARCHITECT analyzer, Abbott Diagnostics). As reported by Kift *et al.* [6], Abbott NGAL assay has an excellent reproducibility, precision, recovery, linearity, and selectivity. In a pilot study using 136 urine samples and 6 calibration standards, NGAL concentrations by research ELISA and the ARCHITECT assay were highly correlated (r = 0.99). In the most representative study, 196 children undergoing CPB were prospectively enrolled and serial urine NGAL concentrations were obtained by ARCHITECT assay [7]. AKI developed in 99 patients, but the diagnosis of AKI using serum creatinine concentration was delayed by 2 - 3 days after CPB.

On the contrary, mean urine NGAL concentrations increased 15-fold within 2 hours, and by 25-fold at 4 and 6 hours after CPB. For the 2-hour urine NGAL concentration, the AUC was 0.95, sensitivity was 0.82, and specificity was 0.90 for the prediction of AKI using a cut-off value of 100 μg/L. The 2-hour urine NGAL levels correlated with severity and duration of AKI, length of stay, dialysis requirement, and death. Thus, non-biased measurements of urine NGAL are obtained using the ARCHITECT platform. Urine NGAL concentration measured by ARCHITECT assay was found to be an early predictive biomarker of AKI severity after CPB [7].

Conclusion

The few studies presented in this chapter are the representatives of growing literature in this field of interest. All the studies seem to support the finding that plasma and/or urine NGAL has a very good diagnostic performance in the early detection of AKI that is a complication of different diseases. NGAL has many of the prerequisites to become one of the most promising next-generation biomarkers for clinical use.

References

[1]   Dent CL, Ma Q, Dastrala S, Bennett M, Mitsnefes MM, Barasch J, Devarajan P. Plasma neutrophil gelatinase-associated lipocalin predicts acute kidney injury, morbidity and mortality after pediatric cardiac surgery: a prospective uncontrolled cohort study. *Crit Care* 2007;11:R127.

[2]   Devarajan P. Neutrophil gelatinase-associated lipocalin (NGAL): A new marker of kidney disease. *Scand J Clin Lab Invest Suppl* 2008;241:89–94.

[3]   Soto K, Papoila AL, Coelho S, Bennett M, Ma Q, Rodrigues B, Fidalgo P, Frade F, Devarajan P. Plasma NGAL for the diagnosis of AKI in patients admitted from the emergency department setting. *Clin J Am Soc Nephrol* 2013;8:2053-63.

[4]   Vijayasimha M, Padma V, Das Mujumdar SK, Satyanarayana P. Evaluation of the diagnostic performance of new markers for acute kidney injury associated with contrast administration. *J Mahatma Gandhi Inst Med Sci* 2013;18:116-21.

[5]   Kim H, Hur M, Cruz DN, Moon HW, Yun YM. Plasma neutrophil gelatinase-associated lipocalin as a biomarker for acute kidney injury in critically ill patients with suspected sepsis *Clin Biochem* 2013;46:1414–8.

[6]   Kift RL, Messenger MP, Wind TC, Hepburn S, Wilson M, Thompson D, Smith MW, Sturgeon C, Lewington AJ, Selby PJ, Banks RE. A comparison of the analytical performance of five commercially available assays for neutrophil gelatinase-associated lipocalin using urine. *Ann Clin Biochem* 2013;50:236-44.

[7]   Bennett M, Dent CL, Ma Q, Dastrala S, Grenier F, Workman R, Syed H, Ali S, Barasch J, Devarajan P. Urine NGAL predicts severity of acute kidney injury after cardiac surgery: a prospective study. *Clin J Am Soc Nephrol* 2008;3:665-73.

In: Neutrophil Gelatinase-Associated Lipocalin   ISBN: 978-1-63117-984-6
Editors: M. Hur and S. Di Somma   © 2014 Nova Science Publishers, Inc.

Chapter 9

Stability and Half-Life: *In Vitro, Preanalytical Factors*

Patrizia Cardelli[*]

Department of Molecular and Clinical Medicine, Sant'Andrea Hospital,
Sapienza University, School of Medicine, Rome, Italy

Abstract

Measurement of a biomarker such as NGAL is an important aid to clinicians in the early detection, diagnosis, monitoring, and prognosis of a pathological condition. Specimen quality plays a key role in assuring the availability of reliable assays in clinical laboratories. In this chapter, the half-life and stability of NGAL are discussed.

Introduction

Normal human plasma contains 72 ng/mL of NGAL (range 40 – 109 ng/mL) in two main forms, monomer and dimer [1]. Axelsson et al. [1] observed, following intravenous injection of 125-iodine labelled NGAL, a more rapid initial clearance of the monomeric form than the dimeric form ($t_{1/2}$

---

[*] Correspondence: patrizia.cardelli@uniroma1.it.

10 min vs. 20 min) and a second phase during which the two NGAL forms were cleared at similar rates.

The Half-Life of NGAL

Plasma NGAL is easily filtered by the glomerulus and reabsorbed in the apical membranes of the proximal tubules. Reabsorption is mediated by megalin-cubulin dependent endocytosis. The delivered iron is needed in processes activating and repressing iron-responsive genes that are vital to the regeneration processes that occur after damage is inflicted to these cells [2]. Under normal circumstances, the estimated half life of plasma NGAL is approximately 10 minutes, with urinary loss less than 0.2% [1-3]. NGAL fulfills a central role in regulating epithelial neogenesis and in iron chelation and delivery after ischemic or toxic insults to the renal tubular epithelium [4, 5].

After kidney injury, NGAL is rapidly expressed on the apical epithelial membranes of the distal nephron. NGAL is excreted in the urine through exocytosis and has local bacteriostatic and proapoptotic effects [6, 7]. Plasma NGAL and urine NGAL concentrations increase by 10- to 100-folds during the 2 hours following tubular injury [8, 9]. On the contrary, serum creatinine does not start to rise until 24 to 72 hours after the initial renal insult [9-11].

Stability of NGAL

NGAL can be measured in different biological fluids including blood and urine. When peripheral blood is used, the suitable fraction for NGAL assay is the plasma; serum must be avoided because NGAL is released from neutrophils during the coagulation process and could result in false pathological increase. In plasma, NGAL is stable for 48 hours at 4°C. Long term storage at -80°C is recommended [12-14], but storage at − 20°C should be avoid.

NGAL in urine is stable at 4°C for up to 7 days [13]. If stored for a long time, a -80°C temperature is required because long-term specimen storage at − 20°C lead to significant and variable changes in urine NGAL concentration [13]. Moreover, several freeze-thaw procedures do not affect the NGAL measurement in plasma or urine samples [12, 13].

As reported by Grenier et al. [13], urine NGAL measured with the CMIA ARCHITET was unaffected when the assay was performed in presence of the following potential interfering endogenous substances: acetone, ascorbic acid, albumin, bilirubin, creatinine, ethanol, glucose, hemoglobin, NaCl, oxalic acid, riboflavin, or urea. Moreover the assay was also insensitive to sample pH ranging from 4 to 9.

Hemolysis can interfere with NGAL measurements in plasma. Pedersen et al. [12] found a direct relationship between degree of hemolysis and NGAL increase, and a high inter-assay variation in urine samples than in plasma samples. They suggested that this difference could be caused by the presence of sedimentation factors in urine, which can influence the assay imprecision. These results underline the importance of centrifugation of urine samples prior to NGAL assay with ELISA methods [15].

In urine samples from patients with urinary tract diseases/infections [16], it is important to take into account the possible production of NGAL by infiltrating neutrophils. Tubular epithelial cells predominantly secrete the monomeric form, while the dimeric form is the predominant form secreted by neutrophils [17]. It means that NGAL is present in different molecular forms in urine; as a consequence, the antibody (antibodies) constructed to recognize renal NGAL may also recognize leukocyte NGAL, having an effect on the clinical performance of the chosen assay [9, 12, 17]. Cai et al. [17] concluded that it should be possible to construct an assay that preferentially identifies NGAL originating from the tubular epithelium or the neutrophils because the molecular structure of NGAL seems slightly different between these two sources. Such an assay should be more specific and sensitive in the detection of AKI and of major benefit for patients at risk of developing impaired kidney function. Indeed, Decavele et al. [18] were able to demonstrate that urinary WBC counts were significantly correlated with urinary NGAL values. The correlation between NGAL and leukocyturia was found for both upper and lower urinary tract infections. They suggested a mathematical correction in cases with pyuria ($> 100 \times 10^9$ cells/L) and urinary NGAL concentration > 100 µg/L.

Conclusion

The rapid kinetics of NGAL is considered of certain usefulness in the diagnostic field of acute illnesses, i.e., acute kidney injury. Moreover, its stability allows the molecule to be reliable in various clinical situations with an optimal sensitivity and specificity. NGAL can be used with acceptable precision, even if hemolysis can affect the diagnostic accuracy of this molecule.

References

[1] Axelsson L, Bergenfeldt M, Ohlsson K. Studies of the release and turnover of a human neutrophil lipocalin. *Scand J Clin Lab Invest* 1995;55:577-88.

[2] de Geus HR, Bakker J, Lesaffre EM, le Noble JL. Neutrophil gelatinase-associated lipocalin at ICU admission predicts for acute kidney injury in adult patients. *Am J Respir Crit Care Med* 2011;183:907-14.

[3] Mori K, Lee HT, Rapoport D, Drexler IR, Foster K, Yang J, Schmidt-Ott KM, Chen X, Li JY, Weiss S, Mishra J, Cheema FH, Markowitz G, Suganami T, Sawai K, Mukoyama M, Kunis C, D'Agati V, Devarajan P, Barasch J. Endocytic delivery of lipocalin-siderophore-iron complex rescues the kidney from ischemia- reperfusion injury. *J Clin Invest* 2005;115:610–21.

[4] Yang J, Goetz D, Li JY, Wang W, Mori K, Setlik D, Du T, Erdjument-Bromage H, Tempst P, Strong R, Barasch J. An iron delivery pathway mediated by a lipocalin. *Mol Cell* 2002;10:1045–56.

[5] Gwira JA, Wei F, Ishiibe S, Ueland JM, Barasch J, Cantley LG. Expression of neutrophil gelatinase-associated lipocalin regulates epithelial morphogenesis in vitro. J *Biol Chem* 2005;280:7875–82.

[6] Schmidt-Ott KM, Mori K, Kalandadze A, Li JY, Paragas N, Nicholas T, Devarajan P, Barasch J. Neutrophil gelatinase-associated lipocalin-mediated iron traffic in kidney epithelia. *Curr Opin Nephrol Hypertens* 2006;15:442–9.

[7] Schmidt-Ott KM, Mori K, Li JY, Kalandadze A, Cohen DJ, Devarajan P, Barasch J. Dual action of neutrophil gelatinase-associated lipocalin. *J Am Soc Nephrol* 2007;18:407–13.

[8] Mishra J, Ma Q, Prada A, Mitsnefes M, Zahedi K, Yang J, Barasch J, Devarajan P. Identification of neutrophil gelatinase-associated lipocalin as a novel early urinary biomarker for ischemic renal injury. *J Am Soc Nephrol* 2003;14:2534–43.

[9] Mishra J, Dent C, Tarabishi R, Mitsnefes MM, Ma Q, Kelly C, Ruff SM, Zahedi K, Shao M, Bean J, Mori K, Barasch J, Devarajan P. Neutrophil

gelatinase-associated lipocalin (NGAL) as a biomarker for acute renal injury after cardiac surgery. *Lancet* 2005;365:1231–8.

[10] Zappitelli M, Washburn KK, Arikan AA, Loftis L, Ma Q, Devarajan P, Parikh CR, Goldstein SL. Urine neutrophil gelatinase-associated lipocalin is an early marker of acute kidney injury in critically ill children: a prospective cohort study. *Crit Care* 2007;11:R84.

[11] Haase-Fielitz A, Bellomo R, Devarajan P, Story D, Matalanis G, Dragun D, Haase M. Novel and conventional serum biomarkers predicting acute kidney injury in adult cardiac surgery: a prospective cohort study. *Crit Care Med* 2009;37:553–60.

[12] Pedersen KR, Ravn HB, Hjortdal VE, Nø rregaard R, Povlsen JV. Neutrophil gelatinase-associated lipocalin (NGAL): validation of commercially available ELISA. *Scand J Clin Lab Invest* 2010;70: 374– 82.

[13] Grenier FC, Ali S, Syed H, Workman R, Martens F, Liao M, Wang Y, Wong PY. Evaluation of the ARCHITECT urine NGAL assay: Assay performance, specimen handling requirements and biological variability. *Clin Biochem* 2010;43:615–20.

[14] Haase-Fielitz A, Haase M, Bellomo R. Instability of urinary NGAL during long-term storage. *Am J Kidney Dis* 2009;53:564–5.

[15] Clerico A, Galli C, Fortunato A, Ronco C. Neutrophil gelatinase-associated lipocalin (NGAL) as biomarker of acute kidney injury: a review of the laboratory characteristics and clinical evidences. *Clin Chem Lab Med* 2012;50:1505-17.

[16] Xu SY, Carlson M, Engström A, Garcia R, Peterson CG, Venge P. Purification and characterization of a human neutrophil lipocalin (HNL) from the secondary granules of human neutrophils. *Scand J Clin Lab Invest* 1994;54:365–76.

[17] Cai L, Rubin J, Han W, Venge P, Xu S. The origin of multiple molecular forms in urine of HNL/NGAL. *Clin J Am Soc Nephrol* 2010;5:2229–35.

[18] Decavele AC, Dhondt L, De Buyzere ML, Delanghe J. Increased urinary neutrophil gelatinase associated lipocalin in urinary tract infections and leukocyturia. *Clin Chem Lab Med* 2011;49:999–1003.

In: Neutrophil Gelatinase-Associated Lipocalin   ISBN: 978-1-63117-984-6
Editors: M. Hur and S. Di Somma   © 2014 Nova Science Publishers, Inc.

Chapter 10

Reference Ranges and Cut-Off Values for the NGAL Assay

Yeo-Min Yun[*]

Department of Laboratory Medicine,
Konkuk University School of Medicine, Seoul, Korea

Abstract

At present, no studies agree on the health-associated reference values for the NGAL assay using blood or urine specimens, which are based on large reference populations with stratification according to age, gender, and ethnicity. However, we use reported normal values as reference ranges in relatively large, apparently healthy subjects as a control group to measure NGAL in blood and urine specimens with a limitation. This chapter describes an overview of reference ranges and cut-off values for NGAL as a biomarker for use in clinical practice.

Introduction

Generally, health-associated reference values are obtained by measuring a particular quantity in a reference individual, which is a person selected for

---

[*] Correspondence: ymyun@kuh.ac.kr.

testing on the basis of well-defined criteria to exclude non-healthy individuals from the reference population [1]. However, at present, no studies agree on the health-associated reference values for the NGAL assay using blood or urine specimens based on large reference populations with stratification according to age, gender, and ethnicity [2]. Some clinical studies reported normal values in relatively large, apparently healthy subjects as a control group to measure NGAL in blood and urine specimens [2]. We could consider these reported normal values reference ranges with a limitation. In this text, we normalized the units for blood and urine NGAL values in the original articles as µg/L as an international standard for the NGAL assay.

Reference Ranges for NGAL Assay

The reference ranges for the NGAL assay reported in studies that measured normal values as a control group in blood samples are summarized in Table 1 [3-5].

Table 1. Reference ranges of blood NGAL assay

Reference	Reference range (ug/L)	Mean value (ug/L) (SD)	Method	Sample	Number (M:F)	Characteristics	Age (yr)
Triage® NGAL Product Insert 2011 [3]	< 153 (90% CI: 142-182)	NA	Triage NGAL Test (POCT)	Whole blood, plasma	125 (99:26)	Apparently healthy individuals	Adults
Xiang et al., 2013 [4]	< 122.57	NA	Immunoassay (Cobas c501 system, Roche)	Serum	454 (218:236)	Healthy donors	21-75 (mean, 45)
Stejskal et al., 2008 [5]	NA	M: 86.3 (43.0) F: 88.9 (38.2)	ELISA, in-house	Serum	136 (53:83)	Non-obese, healthy individuals	Adults

Abbreviations: NGAL, neutrophil gelatinase-associated lipocalin; CI, confidence interval; SD, standard deviation; NA, not available; M, male; F, female; yr, years.

The expected normal values reported by the manufacturer could also be used for method-specific reference ranges. On the product label for the Triage NGAL Test (Alere San Diego, Inc., CA, USA), which is reported by the manufacturer to measure NGAL levels in plasma (collecting EDTA blood samples) from 125 apparently healthy subjects (99 males and 26 females), the upper limit (95th percentile) of the non-parametric reference range was 153 µg/L (90% confidence interval [CI], 142 – 182 µg/L) [3].

The study that measured serum NGAL levels using a particle-enhanced turbidimetric immunoassay on the Cobas c501 system (Roche Diagnostics, Germany) reported the upper limit of the reference range to be 122.57 µg/L, based on the 95th percentile of NGAL values measured in 454 healthy donors [4]. In a study that measured serum NGAL levels using a manual ELISA method [5], the mean NGAL value was 86.3 µg/L (SD, 43.0 µg/L; median, 78.8 µg/L) and 88.9 µg/L (SD, 38.2 µg/L; median, 80.0 µg/L) in 53 healthy, non-obese men and 83 healthy, non-obese women, respectively (Table 1).

The reference ranges of the NGAL assay from studies that measured normal values in urine samples are summarized in Table 2 [6 - 11]. The upper limit (95th percentile) of the reference range in urine samples was less than or equal to 131.7 µg/L for the chemiluminescent microparticle immunoassay (CMIA, ARCHITECT Urine NGAL, Abbott Diagnostics, IL, USA) by the manufacturer [6]. The expected range was determined by testing urine samples from 196 non-hospitalized donors that had blood creatinine values within 0.7 and 1.5 mg/dL, and urine protein/urine creatinine ratios less than or equal to 200 mg/g [6].

Cut-Off Values for NGAL Assay

The diagnostic accuracy of the NGAL assay for blood and urine samples to predict the development of acute kidney injury (AKI) in various clinical conditions is summarized in Tables 3 and 4. The data showed various cut-off values with large differences in diagnostic accuracy, with area under the curve (AUC) values ranging from 0.54 to 0.96 for NGAL in blood samples (Table 3) [12-25], and from 0.61 to 0.98 in urine samples (Table 4) [14-16, 18, 22, 24, 26-36].

In some studies, NGAL assays showed a relatively good discriminate power to predict AKI development, whereas in other studies, NGAL assays were very poor at or could not distinguish patients with or without AKI [2].

Table 2. Reference ranges of urinary NGAL assay

Reference	Upper limit of reference range (ug/L)	Mean value (ug/L) (SD)	Method	Sample	Number (M:F)	Characteristics	Age (yr)
ARCHITECT Urine NGAL Product Insert 2009 [6]	131.7	NA	CMIA (Architect, Abbott)	Urine	196	Non-hospitalized donors that had blood Cr values of 0.7 to 1.5 mg/dL and urine protein/urine Cr ratios ≤ 200 mg/g	NA
Schinstock et al. 2013 [7]	M: 65 (52.2-75.7) F: 23.4 (17.1-29.7)	NA	ELISA (BioPorto Diagnostics)	24h urine	125 (58:67)	Normal volunteers	22-77 (mean, 45.7)
Pennemans et al. 2013 [8]	M/F (95th percentile) 0-10 yrs: 52.97/141.80 11-20 yrs: 62.50/145.43 21-30 yrs: 73.88/149.29 31-40 yrs: 87.54/153.60 41-50 yrs: 103.95/158.37 51-60 yrs: 123.7/163.62 61-70 yrs: 146.52/169.38 71-80 yrs: 176.31/175.68 >81 yrs: 211.16/182.58	NA	ELISA (R&D Systems)	Urine	338 (139:199)	Healthy, non-smoking adults (exclusion of 12% by criteria)	0-95 (mean, 45.8)
Cangemi et al. 2013 [9]	97.5th percentile: 58.7 99th percentile: 109.4	10.2 (17.5)	CMIA (Architect, Abbott)	Urine	308	Healthy children	Neonates–children
Huynh et al. 2009 [10]	95th percentile (CI) All: 50 (33.9-82.2) M: 20 (16.9-26.0)	All: 5 (4.7-5.4) M: 5 (4.8-	Immunoblot, in-house	Urine	50 (30:20)	Very low birth weight infants	Infants

Reference	Upper limit of reference range (ug/L)	Mean value (ug/L) (SD)	Method	Sample	Number (M:F)	Characteristics	Age (yr)
	F: 100 (83.5-116.3)	5.2) F: 10 (9.0-11.1)					
Rybi-Szuminska et al. 2013 [11]	Age: NGAL/Cr ratio 0.2-5.9: 33.91 ng/mg 6-9.9: 26.23 ng/mg 10-13.9: 20.29 ng/mg 14-17.9: 15.69 ng/mg	NA	ELISA (R&D Systems)	Urine	172 (88:84)	Healthy children and adolescents	0.2-17.9 (median, 9.75)

Abbreviations: NGAL, neutrophil gelatinase-associated lipocalin; CI, confidence interval; M, male; F, female; SD, standard deviation; NA, not available; CMIA, Chemiluminescent microparticle immunoassay; Cr, creatinine.

Table 3. Cutoff values of blood NGAL assay

Reference	Clinical setting	Cutoff value (ug/L)	AKI diagnosis	Method	Sample	Sampling time	Sensitivity (%)	Specificity (%)	AUC (95% CI)	PPV	NPV	N (N of AKI)
Haase-Fielitz et al. 2009[12]	CS	150	Cr increase of 50% or > 0.3 mg/dL	Triage	Serum	ICU arrival	79	78	0.80 (0.63 – 0.96)	0.52	0.93	100 (23)
Koyner et al. 2008 [13]	CS	NA	Cr increase of 50% or > 0.3 mg/dL	ELISA	Plasma	immediately after CPB, 6 h after ICU arrival	NA	NA	0.54 (0.40– 0.67)	NA	NA	72 (34)

Table 3. (Continued)

Reference	Clinical setting	Cutoff value (ug/L)	AKI diagnosis	Method	Sample	Sampling time	Sensitivity (%)	Specificity (%)	AUC (95% CI)	PPV	NPV	N (N of AKI)
Parikh et al. 2011 [14]	CS	293	Acute dialysis or 2-fold Cr increase	Triage	Plasma	0-6 h after ICU arrival	50	82	0.70	NA	NA	1,219 (71)
Tuladhar et al. 2009 [15]	CS	426	Cr increase > 0.5 mg/dL	ELISA	Plasma	Preoperative, 2 h after CPB	80	66.7	0.85 (0.73 – 0.97)	NA	NA	50 (9)
Mishra et al. 2005 [16]	CS (P)	25	50% Cr increase	ELISA	Serum	2 h after CPB	70	94	0.91	0.82	0.89	71 (20)
Dent et al. 2007 [17]	CS (P)	150	50 % Cr increase	Triage	Plasma	2 h after CPB	84	94	0.96 (0.94-0.99)	0.84	0.93	120 (45)
Parikh et al. 2011[18]	CS (P)	154	Acute dialysis or 2-fold Cr increase	Triage	Plasma	0 - 6 h after ICU arrival	59	54	0.56	0.20	0.86	311 (53)
Cruz et al. 2010 [19]	IC	150	50 % Cr increase	Triage	Plasma	Within 4 days after ICU admission	73	81	0.78 (0.65 – 0.90)	24	97	301 (133)
Constantin et al. 2010 [20]	IC	155	50 % Cr increase	Triage	Plasma	2 h after ICU arrival	82	97	0.92 (0.85 – 0.97)	97	80	56 (20)
Wheeler et al. 2008	IC (P)	139	BUN > 100 mg/dL,	ELISA	Serum	24 h after ICU arrival	86	39	0.68 (0.56 –	39	94	143 (22)

Reference	Clinical setting	Cutoff value (ug/L)	AKI diagnosis	Method	Sample	Sampling time	Sensitivity (%)	Specificity (%)	AUC (95% CI)	PPV	NPV	N (N of AKI)
[21]			Cr> 2 mg/dL or need for dialysis						0.79)			
Portal et al. 2010 [22]	LT	258	2–3-fold Cr increase	ELISA	Plasma	Within 24 h of LT	74	85	0.87 (0.77 – 0.93)	NA	NA	80 (30)
Niemann et al. 2009 [23]	LT	NA	50% Cr increase	ELISA	Serum	Immediately after anesthetic induction, 2h and 24h after reperfusion	68	80	0.79	NA	NA	45 (24)
Hirsch et al. 2007 [24]	CM (P)	100	50% Cr increase	ELISA	Plasma	2h after contrast administration	73	100	0.91	NA	NA	91 (11)
Malyszko et al. 2009 [25]	CM	> 25% increase	25% Cr increase	ELISA	Serum	Preoperative, 2, 4, 8, 24, 48 h after CPB	90	74	NR	NA	NA	140 (70)

Abbreviations: NGAL, neutrophil gelatinase-associated lipocalin; AKI, acute kidney injury; AUC, area under the curve; CI, confidence interval; PPV, positive predictive value; NPV, negative predictive value; N, number; SD, standard deviation; NA, not available; Cr, creatinine; CS, cardiac surgery; P, pediatric; ICU, intensive care unit; CM, contrast medium; LT, liver transplant; CPB, cardiopulmonary bypass.

Table 4. Cutoff values of urinary NGAL assay

Reference	Clinical setting	Cutoff value (ug/L)	AKI diagnosis	Method	Sampling time	Sensitivity (%)	Specificity (%)	AUC (95% CI)	PPV	NPV	N (AKI developed)
Wagener et al. 2008 [26]	CS[a]	65	Cr increase> 0.5 mg/dL	ELISA	18 h after CS	NA	NA	0.61 (0.54-0.68)	NA	NA	426 (85)
Parikh et al. 2011 [14]	CS	102	Acute dialysis or 2-fold Cr increase	ARCHITECT	0-6 h after ICU admission	46	81	0.67	NA	NA	1,219 (71)
Wagener et al. 2006 [27]	CS	213	50% Cr increase	Immunoblot	18 h after CS	73	78	0.80 (0.57-1.03)	47	91	81 (16)
Xin et al. 2008 [28]	CS	250	50% Cr increase	ELISA	2 h after CS	71	73	0.88	58	91	33 (9)
Tuladhar et al. 2009 [15]	CS	393	Cr increase > 0.5 mg/dL	ELISA	2 h after CS	93	78	0.96 (0.90-1.0)	NA	NA	50 (9)
Koyner et al. 2010 [29]	CS	NA	Cr increase of 50 % or > 0.3 mg/dL	ELISA	6 h after ICU admission	NA	NA	0.78 (0.61-0.96)	NA	NA	123 (46)
Parikh et al. 2011 [18]	CS (P)	17	Acute dialysis or 2-fold Cr increase	ARCHITECT	6 h after ICU admission	75	65	0.71	30	93	311 (53)
Mishra et al. 2005 [16]	CS (P)	25 or 50	50% Cr increase	ELISA	2 h after CS	100	98	0.99	0.95	1.00	71 (20)
Bennett et al. 2008 [30]	CS (P)	100	50% Cr increase	ELISA	2 h after CS	82	90	0.93	NA	NA	196 (99)

Reference	Clinical setting	Cutoff value (ug/L)	AKI diagnosis	Method	Sampling time	Sensitivity (%)	Specificity (%)	AUC (95% CI)	PPV	NPV	N (AKI developed)
Makris et al. 2009 [31]	IC	25	50% Cr increase or >25% eGFR decrease	ELISA	Immediately after ICU admission	91	95	0.98 (0.82-0.98)	NA	NA	31 (11)
Siew et al. 2009 [32]	IC	NA	Cr increase of 50% or > 0.3 mg/dL	ELISA	24 h after ICU admission	NA	NA	0.71 (0.63-0.78)	NA	NA	451 (86)
Zappitelli et al. 2007 [33]	IC (P)	0.2	eCCl decrease by 25% from baseline	ELISA	Daily (48 h before AKI development)	77	72	0.78 (0.62-0.95)	NA	NA	150 (106)
Ling et al. 2008 [34]	CM	9.85	25% Cr increase	ELISA	2 h after CAG	77	71	0.73 (0.54-0.93)	NA	NA	40 (13)
Hirsch et al. 2007 [24]	CM (P)	100	50% Cr increase	ELISA	2 h after CS	73	100	0.92	100	96	91 (11)
Portal et al. 2010 [22]	LT	150	2 - 3- fold Cr increase	ELISA	Within 12 h of ICU arrival	NA	NA	0.76 (0.60-0.91)	NA	NA	80 (30)
Wagener et al. 2011 [35]	LT	0.74 (uNGAL/uCr)	50% Cr increase	ELISA	3 h after reperfusion	83.5	67.5	0.80 (0.73-0.87)	NA	NA	92 (37)
Nickolas et al. 2008 [36]	EU	85	1.5-fold Cr increase or > 25% eGFR decrease	Immunoblot	NA	90	99.5	0.95 (0.88-1.0)	0.74	1.00	635 (30)

Abbreviations: NGAL, neutrophil gelatinase-associated lipocalin; AKI, acute kidney injury; AUC, area under the curve; CI, confidence interval; PPV, positive predictive value; NPV, negative predictive value; N, number; SD, standard deviation; NA, not available; CS, cardiac surgery; P, pediatric; IC, intensive care; CM, contrast medium; LT, liver transplant; EU, emergency unit; Cr, creatinine; eGFR, estimated glomerular filtration rate; eCCl, estimated creatinine clearance; ICU, intensive care unit;CAG, coronary angiography.

Recently, Hasse et al. [37] reported a systemic review and meta-analysis that evaluated the accuracy of NGAL assays for both the diagnosis and prognosis of AKI. They analyzed data from 19 studies and analyzed 2,538 patients, including 487 (19.2%) patients with AKI. In this study, the overall (487 events/2,538 patients) diagnostic odds ratio and AUC of NGAL to predict AKI development was 18.6 (95% CI, 9.0 – 38.1) and 0.815 (95% CI, 0.732 – 0.892), respectively, with a cut-off value of 190.2 µg/L (95% CI, 122.8 – 257.8 µg/L) [37].

Conclusion

The NGAL assay can be used to predict or diagnose AKI in various clinical settings. The data are, however, still lacking for agreement on reliable reference ranges and cut-off values to predict AKI development in such settings [2]. Further studies are needed to formulate guidelines or recommendations to accurately evaluate NGAL assay reference values in blood and urine samples from reference individuals, which are selected on the basis of well-defined criteria to exclude non-healthy individuals from the reference population [1].

References

[1]   How to Define and Determine Reference Intervals in the Clinical Laboratory; Approved Guideline - Second Edition. In: *Document C28-A2. Wayne,* Pennsylvania: Clinical and Laboratory Standards Institute, 2000.

[2]   Clerico A, Galli C, Fortunato A, Ronco C. Neutrophil gelatinase-associated lipocalin (NGAL) as biomarker of acute kidney injury: a review of the laboratory characteristics and clinical evidences. *Clin Chem Lab Med* 2012;50:1505-17.

[3]   *Triage® NGAL Product Insert.* San Diego, California: Alere San Diego, Inc.; 2011.

[4]   Xiang D, Zhang H, Bai J, Ma J, Li M, Gao W, Zhang X, Gao J, Wang C. Particle-enhanced turbidimetric immunoassay for determination of serum neutrophil gelatinase-associated lipocalin on the Roche Cobas c501 analyzer. *Clin Biochem* 2013;46:1756-60.

[5]   Stejskal D, Karpísek M, Humenanska V, Hanulova Z, Stejskal P, Kusnierova P, Petzel M. Lipocalin-2: development, analytical characterization, and clinical testing of a new ELISA. *Horm Metab Res* 2008;40:381-5.

[6]   *ARCHITECT Urine NGAL Product Insert.* Abbott Park, Illinois, U.S.A.: Abbott Laboratories; 2009.

[7]   Schinstock CA, Semret MH, Wagner SJ, Borland TM, Bryant SC, Kashani KB, Larson TS, Lieske JC. Urinalysis is more specific and urinary neutrophil gelatinase-associated lipocalin is more sensitive for early detection of acute kidney injury. *Nephrol Dial Transplant* 2013;28:1175-85.

[8]   Pennemans V, Rigo JM, Faes C, Reynders C, Penders J, Swennen Q. Establishment of reference values for novel urinary biomarkers for renal damage in the healthy population: are age and gender an issue? *Clin Chem Lab Med* 2013;51:1795-802.

[9]   Cangemi G, Storti S, Cantinotti M, Fortunato A, Emdin M, Bruschettini M, Bugnone D, Melioli G, Clerico A. Reference values for urinary neutrophil gelatinase-associated lipocalin (NGAL) in pediatric age measured with a fully automated chemiluminescent platform. *Clin Chem Lab Med* 2013;51:1101-5.

[10]   Huynh TK, Bateman DA, Parravicini E, Lorenz JM, Nemerofsky SL, Sise ME, Bowman TM, Polesana E, Barasch JM. Reference values of urinary neutrophil gelatinase-associated lipocalin in very low birth weight infants. *Pediatr Res* 2009;66:528-32.

[11]   Rybi-Szuminska A, Wasilewska A, Litwin M, Kulaga Z, Szuminski M. Paediatric normative data for urine NGAL/creatinine ratio. *Acta Paediatr* 2013;102:e269-72.

[12]   Haase-Fielitz A, Bellomo R, Devarajan P, Story D, Matalanis G, Dragun D, Haase M. Novel and conventional serum biomarkers predicting acute kidney injury in adult cardiac surgery--a prospective cohort study. *Crit Care Med* 2009;37:553-60.

[13]   Koyner JL, Bennett MR, Worcester EM, Ma Q, Raman J, Jeevanandam V, Kasza KE, O'Connor MF, Konczal DJ, Trevino S, Devarajan P, Murray PT. Urinary cystatin C as an early biomarker of acute kidney injury following adult cardiothoracic surgery. *Kidney Int* 2008;74:1059-69.

[14]   Parikh CR, Coca SG, Thiessen-Philbrook H, Shlipak MG, Koyner JL, Wang Z, Edelstein CL, Devarajan P, Patel UD, Zappitelli M, Krawczeski CD, Passik CS, Swaminathan M, Garg AX; TRIBE-AKI

Consortium. Postoperative biomarkers predict acute kidney injury and poor outcomes after adult cardiac surgery. *J Am Soc Nephrol* 2011;22:1748-57.

[15] Tuladhar SM, Puntmann VO, Soni M, Punjabi PP, Bogle RG. Rapid detection of acute kidney injury by plasma and urinary neutrophil gelatinase-associated lipocalin after cardiopulmonary bypass. *J Cardiovasc Pharmacol* 2009;53:261-6.

[16] Mishra J, Dent C, Tarabishi R, Mitsnefes MM, Ma Q, Kelly C, Ruff SM, Zahedi K, Shao M, Bean J, Mori K, Barasch J, Devarajan P. Neutrophil gelatinase-associated lipocalin (NGAL) as a biomarker for acute renal injury after cardiac surgery. *Lancet* 2005;365:1231-8.

[17] Dent CL, Ma Q, Dastrala S, Bennett M, Mitsnefes MM, Barasch J, Devarajan P. Plasma neutrophil gelatinase-associated lipocalin predicts acute kidney injury, morbidity and mortality after pediatric cardiac surgery: a prospective uncontrolled cohort study. *Crit Care* 2007;11:R127.

[18] Parikh CR, Devarajan P, Zappitelli M, Sint K, Thiessen-Philbrook H, Li S, Kim RW, Koyner JL, Coca SG, Edelstein CL, Shlipak MG, Garg AX, Krawczeski CD; TRIBE-AKI Consortium. Postoperative biomarkers predict acute kidney injury and poor outcomes after pediatric cardiac surgery. *J Am Soc Nephrol* 2011;22:1737-47.

[19] Cruz DN, de Cal M, Garzotto F, Perazella MA, Lentini P, Corradi V, Piccinni P, Ronco C. Plasma neutrophil gelatinase-associated lipocalin is an early biomarker for acute kidney injury in an adult ICU population. *Intensive Care Med* 2010;36:444-51.

[20] Constantin JM, Futier E, Perbet S, Roszyk L, Lautrette A, Gillart T, Guerin R, Jabaudon M, Souweine B, Bazin JE, Sapin V. Plasma neutrophil gelatinase-associated lipocalin is an early marker of acute kidney injury in adult critically ill patients: a prospective study. *J Crit Care* 2010;25:176.e1-6.

[21] Wheeler DS, Devarajan P, Ma Q, Harmon K, Monaco M, Cvijanovich N, Wong HR. Serum neutrophil gelatinase-associated lipocalin (NGAL) as a marker of acute kidney injury in critically ill children with septic shock. *Crit Care Med* 2008;36:1297-303.

[22] Portal AJ, McPhail MJ, Bruce M, Coltart I, Slack A, Sherwood R, Heaton ND, Shawcross D, Wendon JA, Heneghan MA. Neutrophil gelatinase--associated lipocalin predicts acute kidney injury in patients undergoing liver transplantation. *Liver Transpl* 2010;16:1257-66.

[23] Niemann CU, Walia A, Waldman J, Davio M, Roberts JP, Hirose R, Feiner J. Acute kidney injury during liver transplantation as determined by neutrophil gelatinase-associated lipocalin. *Liver Transpl* 2009;15:1852-60.

[24] Hirsch R, Dent C, Pfriem H, Allen J, Beekman RH 3rd, Ma Q, Dastrala S, Bennett M, Mitsnefes M, Devarajan P. NGAL is an early predictive biomarker of contrast-induced nephropathy in children. *Pediatr Nephrol* 2007;22:2089-95.

[25] Malyszko J, Bachorzewska-Gajewska H, Poniatowski B, Malyszko JS, Dobrzycki S. Urinary and serum biomarkers after cardiac catheterization in diabetic patients with stable angina and without severe chronic kidney disease. *Ren Fail* 2009;31:910-9.

[26] Wagener G, Gubitosa G, Wang S, Borregaard N, Kim M, Lee HT. Urinary neutrophil gelatinase-associated lipocalin and acute kidney injury after cardiac surgery. *Am J Kidney Dis* 2008;52:425-33.

[27] Wagener G, Jan M, Kim M, Mori K, Barasch JM, Sladen RN, Lee HT. Association between increases in urinary neutrophil gelatinase-associated lipocalin and acute renal dysfunction after adult cardiac surgery. *Anesthesiology* 2006;105:485-91.

[28] Xin C, Yulong X, Yu C, Changchun C, Feng Z, Xinwei M. Urine neutrophil gelatinase-associated lipocalin and interleukin-18 predict acute kidney injury after cardiac surgery. *Ren Fail* 2008;30:904-13.

[29] Koyner JL, Vaidya VS, Bennett MR, Ma Q, Worcester E, Akhter SA, Raman J, Jeevanandam V, O'Connor MF, Devarajan P, Bonventre JV, Murray PT. Urinary biomarkers in the clinical prognosis and early detection of acute kidney injury. *Clin J Am Soc Nephrol* 2010;5:2154-65.

[30] Bennett M, Dent CL, Ma Q, Dastrala S, Grenier F, Workman R, Syed H, Ali S, Barasch J, Devarajan P. Urine NGAL predicts severity of acute kidney injury after cardiac surgery: a prospective study. *Clin J Am Soc Nephrol* 2008;3:665-73.

[31] Makris K, Markou N, Evodia E, Dimopoulou E, Drakopoulos I, Ntetsika K, Rizos D, Baltopoulos G, Haliassos A. Urinary neutrophil gelatinase-associated lipocalin (NGAL) as an early marker of acute kidney injury in critically ill multiple trauma patients. *Clin Chem Lab Med* 2009;47:79-82.

[32] Siew ED, Ware LB, Gebretsadik T, Shintani A, Moons KG, Wickersham N, Bossert F, Ikizler TA. Urine neutrophil gelatinase-

associated lipocalin moderately predicts acute kidney injury in critically ill adults. *J Am Soc Nephrol* 2009;20:1823-32.

[33] Zappitelli M, Washburn KK, Arikan AA, Loftis L, Ma Q, Devarajan P, Parikh CR, Goldstein SL. Urine neutrophil gelatinase-associated lipocalin is an early marker of acute kidney injury in critically ill children: a prospective cohort study. *Crit Care* 2007;11:R84.

[34] Ling W, Zhaohui N, Ben H, Leyi G, Jianping L, Huili D, Jiaqi Q. Urinary IL-18 and NGAL as early predictive biomarkers in contrast-induced nephropathy after coronary angiography. *Nephron Clin Pract* 2008;108:c176-81.

[35] Wagener G, Minhaz M, Mattis FA, Kim M, Emond JC, Lee HT. Urinary neutrophil gelatinase-associated lipocalin as a marker of acute kidney injury after orthotopic liver transplantation. *Nephrol Dial Transplant* 2011;26:1717-23.

[36] Nickolas TL, O'Rourke MJ, Yang J, Sise ME, Canetta PA, Barasch N, Buchen C, Khan F, Mori K, Giglio J, Devarajan P, Barasch J. Sensitivity and specificity of a single emergency department measurement of urinary neutrophil gelatinase-associated lipocalin for diagnosing acute kidney injury. *Ann Intern Med* 2008;148:810-9.

[37] Haase M, Bellomo R, Devarajan P, Schlattmann P, Haase-Fielitz A. Accuracy of neutrophil gelatinase-associated lipocalin (NGAL) in diagnosis and prognosis in acute kidney injury: a systematic review and meta-analysis. *Am J Kidney Dis* 2009;54:1012-24.

In: Neutrophil Gelatinase-Associated Lipocalin   ISBN: 978-1-63117-984-6
Editors: M. Hur and S. Di Somma   © 2014 Nova Science Publishers, Inc.

Chapter 11

NGAL vs. Creatinine

Hee-Won Moon and Mina Hur[*]

Department of Laboratory Medicine,
Konkuk University School of Medicine, Seoul, Korea

Abstract

Serum creatinine has been used to assess renal function and renal injury. Serum creatinine increases after considerable loss of kidney function, and the subsequent delay in detection and management may cause irreversible renal damages. Serum creatinine is affected by age, gender, exercise, and nutritional status, which make accurate assessment of renal function difficult.

Thus, ideal biomarkers other than creatinine are needed for accurate assessment of renal function and early detection of acute kidney injury (AKI). Neutrophil gelatinase-associated lipocalin (NGAL) is considered a reliable diagnostic and prognostic biomarker for AKI. This chapter describes an overview of creatinine including its conventional use and limitations in comparison with NGAL.

[*] Correspondence: dearmina@hanmail.net.

Introduction

Acute kidney injury (AKI) represents an abrupt loss of kidney function occurring over the course of hours to days. AKI is common in critical care and perioperative settings, with the reported incidence of 5% to 7% in hospitalized patients and up to 25% in critically ill patients [1]. The spectrum of AKI ranges from a minimal elevation of serum creatinine to anuric renal failure [2, 3]. In spite of improved clinical outcomes, the mortality rate of AKI is still high, ranging from 28% to 90% [4].

Serum creatinine and urine output are commonly used to assess renal function and injury. Creatinine level increases only after the kidney function is considerably lost, and the delay in detection subsequently means the delay in appropriate management, which can cause irreversible renal damages [5]. Serum creatinine also has several limitations, which make accurate assessment of renal function difficult. Thus, ideal biomarkers other than creatinine are needed for the accurate assessment of renal function and early detection of AKI [3, 6 - 8].

From a laboratory point of view, an ideal biomarker should be measured non-invasively, rapid, inexpensive, and amendable to standardized laboratory platforms [1, 5]. Among the potential biomarkers, neutrophil gelatinase-associated lipocalin (NGAL) is considered the most reliable biomarker for AKI, and it can be measured using automated assays [6, 9, 10]. Useful biomarkers show differences in the spectrum of AKI. In the early phase of kidney injury, damage biomarkers such as NGAL may increase, while functional biomarkers such as creatinine remain normal. In the later phase, functional biomarkers increase due to a significant decrease in glomerular filtration rate (GFR) (Figure 1).

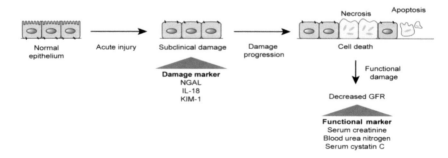

Figure 1. The spectrum of acute kidney injury. Modified by permission from De Gruyter Ltd: [Clinical Chemistry and Laboratory Medicine] [5], copyright (2012).

Creatinine

Creatinine is produced mainly from metabolism of creatine and phsphocreatine in muscle [11, 12]. Creatine is synthesized in the kidneys, liver, and pancreas by enzymatic reactions, in which transamidation of arginine, formation of guanidinoacetic acid, and methylation of guanidinoacetic acid subsequently occur. Creatine is phosphorylated to phosphocreatine, a high-energy compound, in the organs such as muscle and brain. During the process of muscle contraction, interconversion of phosphocreatine and creatine occurs, and small proportion of free creatine in muscle spontaneously converts to creatinine (Figure 2).

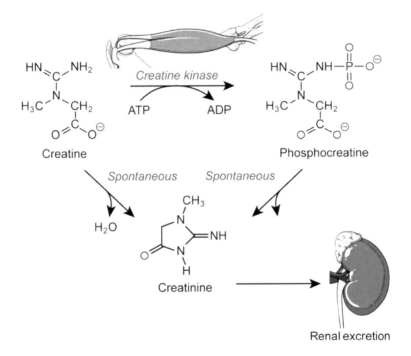

Figure 2. Creatine metabolism and synthesis of creatinine.

Creatinine is freely filtered at the glomerulus, and its concentration is inversely related to the GFR. However, there is a non-linear reciprocal relationship between serum creatinine and GFR, thus making creatinine level insensitive to mild to moderate reduction of GFR (Figure 3) [11]. Serum creatinine remains within the reference interval until renal function is considerably lost (> 50%) [4, 6, 13, 14]. Serum creatinine measurement will fail to detect patients with stage 2 chronic kidney disease (CKD) (GFR, 60 to 89 mL/min/1.73 m²) and many patients with stage 3 CKD (GFR, 30 to 59 mL/min/1.73 m²). In patients with CKD, extrarenal clearance of creatinine occurs in the small intestine by degradation due to bacterial overgrowth, and it could blunt the increase of serum creatinine [15]. Thus, normal serum creatinine does not rule out abnormal kidney function.

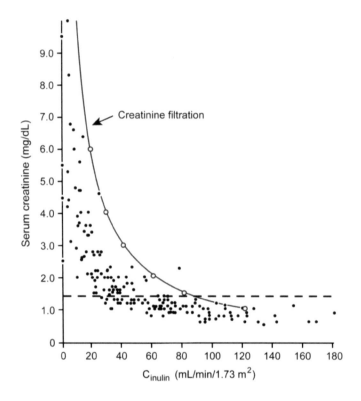

Figure 3. Serum creatinine level vs. glomerular filtration rate (GFR), measured as the clearance of inulin, in 171 patients with glomerular disease. A continuous line represents hypothetical relationship between GFR and serum creatinine, assuming that creatinine is excreted solely by glomerular filtration. The broken horizontal line represents the upper limit of a normal serum creatinine in this study (1.4 mg/dL). Adapted by permission from Macmillan Publishers Ltd: [Kidney International] [14], copyright (1985).

    The reference interval of serum creatinine reflects the range of muscle mass in the reference population studied [11, 12]. It is also affected by age, gender, exercise, and nutritional status [13, 16]. Moreover, a small proportion (7 - 10%) of creatinine in urine is derived from tubular secretion, which is increased in the presence of renal insufficiency [17]. Several medications (e.g., cimetidine, trimethoprim) inhibit the tubular secretion and increase serum creatinine concentrations [4, 11]. Moreover, serum creatinine cannot distinguish pre-renal AKI from renal and post- renal AKI [18].

Creatinine can be measured using chemical and enzymatic methods. The Jaffe reaction (alkaline picrate methods) is the most commonly used chemical method. The Jaffe reaction, however, is not specific for creatinine and subject to interference due to Jaffe-like chromogens, including protein, glucose, ascorbic acid, ketone bodies, pyruvate, guanidine, hemoglobin F, blood-substitute products, and cephalosporins [16, 19, 20]. Enzymatic methods involve a multistep approach leading to a photometric equilibrium and show less interference than the Jaffe methods. However, bilirubin, metamizol, 5-fluorocytosine, dopamine, dobutamine, O-raffinose cross-linked hemoglobin, and monoclonal IgM can interfere with the enzymatic methods [21, 22]. High-performance liquid chromatography (HPLC) procedures and isotope-dilution mass spectrometry (IDMS) methods have been developed, and gas chromatography–IDMS (GC-IDMS) is now considered the method of choice for the creatinine measurement [21, 22]. The Jaffe reaction produces a positive bias by up to 20% compared with HPLC or IDMS methods at physiologic concentrations [13, 23, 24].

Estimation of GFR

The nonlinear relationship between creatinine level and GFR can be corrected using various equations, and the Modification of Diet in Renal Disease (MDRD) study equation, developed in 1999, has been used widely [25]. Although the MDRD equation provides a reliable result using readily available data, there is a significant negative bias and poor precision at higher values of GFR [26]. Thus, numeric values of GFR should be reported only up to 60 mL/min/1.73 m^2 using the MDRD equation [21]. In 2009, the Chronic Kidney Disease Epidemiology Collaboration (CKD-EPI) has suggested a new equation as below [27].

The CKD-EPI equation is less biased than the MDRD equation, and it has been suggested that the CKD-EPI equation should replace the MDRD equation for clinical use [27]. Kidney Disease: Improving Global Outcomes (KDIGO) 2012 clinical practice guideline for the evaluation and management of CKD recommends that clinicians use a GFR-estimating equation to derive GFR from serum creatinine (eGFR$_{creat}$) rather than relying on the serum creatinine concentration alone. It also recommends that clinical laboratories should measure serum creatinine using a specific assay with calibration traceable to the international standard reference materials and minimal bias compared to IDMS reference methodology and report eGFR$_{creat}$ using the 2009 CKD-EPI creatinine equation in adults in addition to the serum creatinine concentration [28]. The estimated GFR levels less than 60 mL/min/1.73 m^2 should be reported as "decreased."

$$GFR = 141 \times \min (Scr/\kappa, 1)^{\alpha} \times \max (Scr/\kappa, 1)^{-1.209} \times 0.993^{Age} \times 1.018 \text{ [if female]} \times 1.159 \text{ [if black]}$$

Scr = serum creatinine
κ = 0.7 for females and 0.9 for males
α = -0.329 for females and -0.411 for males
min = the minimum of Scr/κ or 1
max = the maximum of Scr/κ or 1

Definition of AKI

For the definition of AKI, the KIDGO AKI guideline harmonized the prior RIFLE (Risk of renal dysfunction, Injury to the kidney, Failure or Loss of kidney function, and End-stage kidney disease) and AKI network (AKIN) criteria [29, 30]. In the RIFLE criteria, AKI was defined based on a ≥ 50% increase in serum creatinine level occurring over 1 - 7 days or the presence of oliguria for more than 6 hours [4]. The AKIN criteria added an absolute increase in serum creatinine level of 0.3 mg/dL and reduced the timeframe for the increase in serum creatinine level to 48 hours [31, 32]. The KIDGO guideline is keeping the absolute increase in serum creatinine level of ≥ 0.3 mg/dL within 48 hours from the AKIN definition, but returning to the 7-day timeframe for the ≥ 50% increase in serum creatinine level [30]. The clinical application of the KIDGO AKI definition could increase the early recognition of AKI [29].

AKI is defined as any of the following (not graded):

- Increase in SCr by ≥ 0.3 mg/dL (≥ 26.5 umol/L) within 48 hours; or
- Increase in SCr to ≥ 1.5 times baseline, which is known or presumed to have occurred within the prior 7 days; or
- Urine volume < 0.5 mL/kg/h for 6 hours

NGAL

NGAL is a ubiquitous 25-kDa protein covalently bound to gelatinase from neutrophils and belongs to the superfamily of lipocalins, which are proteins specialized in binding and transporting small hydrophobic molecules with β-barrel calyx structure [33-35] (Figure 4).

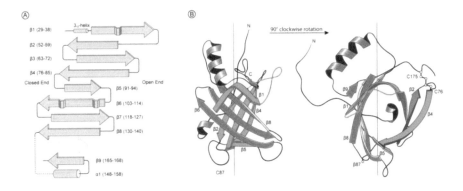

Figure 4. Structure of NGAL. A, schematic representation of the lipocalin fold. The common characteristic of lipocalins is the "lipocalin fold", which comprises an N-terminal 3-10 helix followed by eight beta sheets arranged in an antiparallel orientation. It is connected to an alpha helix and a C-terminal beta sheet. The beta sheets are connected by loops, which form the open end of the molecule (ligand binding site of NGAL). B, Ribbon plots of NGAL. The open end of the barrel is at the right in the left view, while the right view represents a 90° clockwise rotation around the vertical axis and looks into the open end of the barrel. The helices are shown in red and the loops in orange. Adapted from Journal of Molecular Biology, 289, Coles M et al. The solution structure and dynamics of human neutrophil gelatinase-associated lipocalin, 139-157, Copyright (1999), with permission from Elsevier.

NGAL binds some ligands such as the siderophores and modulates most of its biological effects [1, 35]. NGAL interacts with specific surface receptors (including the 24p3R and the megalin multi-scavenger complex) and are present as a complex with iron-siderophores (holo-NGAL) or alone (apo-NGAL). After internalization, holo-NGAL is captured inside endosome and releases the siderophore-iron complex, thus regulating iron-dependent gene pathways. Apo-NGAL conversely captures intra-cellular iron and exports it to the extracellular space (Figure 5) [36]. This process results in depletion of iron reserves and may lead to apoptosis. In this way, NGAL mediates an innate immune response to bacterial infection and may promote cellular apoptosis under particular conditions [37]. NGAL also has other complex activities by interactions with several other receptors and ligands [1, 36, 38].

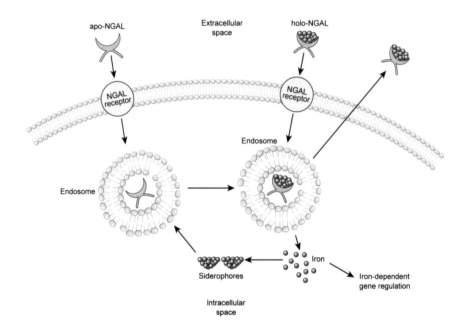

Figure 5. Schematic representation of NGAL-mediated iron traffic. Modified by permission from De Gruyter Ltd: [Clinical Chemistry and Laboratory Medicine] [5], copyright (2012).

NGAL is normally expressed at low level in a variety of human tissues including kidney, trachea, lungs, and colon [33, 34]. The expression of NGAL is upregulated up to 1,000 folds in response to renal tubular injury, thus NGAL has emerged as an early biomarker of renal injury [34]. It is also known that NGAL is markedly induced in a number of human cancers and often represents a predictor of poor prognosis [39, 40].

Plasma NGAL is freely filtered by the glomerulus and largely reabsorbed in the proximal tubules by efficient megalin-dependent endocytosis. Accordingly, urinary excretion of NGAL occurs in conditions of proximal renal tubular injury or increased *de novo* synthesis of NGAL [36]. In AKI, mRNA expression of NGAL is increased in distant organs, especially in liver and lungs. Over-expressed NGAL protein is released into the circulation, and subsequently it results in an increase of plasma NGAL. Furthermore, decreased GFR also cause decreased renal clearance of NGAL [1, 36].

Table 1. Comparison of basic characteristics between creatinine and NGAL

	Creatinine	NGAL
Molecular size	113 Da	25 kDa
Source	Endogenous	Endogenous
Organ	Mainly muscle mass	Various human tissues at low level
Biomarker for	Glomerular filtration	Renal injury
Increase after the renal insult	Several days	2 - 6 hours
Analytical method	Chemical method	ELISA
	Enzyme method	CMIA
	HPLC, GC-IDMS	Point-of-care test
Specific to intrinsic AKI (versus pre-renal)	No	Yes
Cost	Inexpensive	Relatively expensive
Limitation	Dependent on muscle mass, age, gender and nutrition	Influenced by chronic kidney diseases, systemic infections, inflammatory conditions, and malignancies
	Influence of some medications	
	Daily variation	
	Variation between assays	

Abbreviations: NGAL, neutrophil gelatinase associated lipocalin; ELISA, enzyme-linked immunosorbent assay; CMIA, chemiluminscent microparticle immunoassay; HPLC, high-performance liquid chromatography; GC-IDMS, gas chromatography-isotope-dilution mass spectrometry; AKI, acute kidney injury.

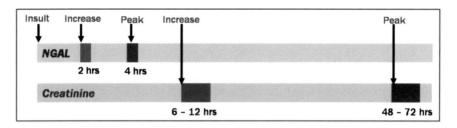

Figure 6. Schematic representation of NGAL and creatinine increases after the renal insult.

NGAL has several limitations as an AKI biomarker. NGAL is not specific to renal tissues, and plasma NGAL can be increased due to damage or altered functional activity of other tissues [41]. Plasma NGAL level can be influenced by various conditions including CKD, hypertension, systemic infections, inflammatory conditions, anemia, hypoxia and malignancies [39, 40, 42, 43]. Although plasma NGAL correlates with the severity of renal impairment in CKD, the increase of plasma NGAL is blunted compared with that typically measured in AKI. Urine NGAL may be also influenced by clinical conditions including CKD, renal inflammation, and urinary tract infection [44 - 46]. Table 1 and Figure 6 show the comparison between creatinine and NGAL.

Conclusion

Creatinine and NGAL are biomarkers with different pathophysiologic properties. Creatinine is a biomarker for kidney function, and NGAL is a marker for AKI. Although NGAL has some limitations and we still lack sufficient data on NGAL, growing evidence has shown that NGAL is a reliable diagnostic and prognostic biomarker for kidney injury. NGAL can detect a subclinical AKI population, which cannot be detected with serum creatinine alone.

References

[1]   Devarajan P. Neutrophil gelatinase-associated lipocalin: a promising biomarker for human acute kidney injury. *Biomark Med* 2010;4:265-80.

[2]   Ronco C, Haapio M, House AA, Anavekar N, Bellomo R. Cardiorenal syndrome. *J Am Coll Cardiol* 2008;52:1527-39.

[3]   Ronco C, McCullough P, Anker SD, Anand I, Aspromonte N, Bagshaw
        SM, Bellomo R, Berl T, Bobek I, Cruz DN, Daliento L, Davenport A,
        Haapio M, Hillege H, House AA, Katz N, Maisel A, Mankad S, Zanco
        P, Mebazaa A, Palazzuoli A, Ronco F, Shaw A, Sheinfeld G, Soni S,
        Vescovo G, Zamperetti N, Ponikowski P; Acute Dialysis Quality
        Initiative (ADQI) consensus group. Cardio-renal syndromes: report from
        the consensus conference of the acute dialysis quality initiative. *Eur
        Heart J* 2010;31:703-11.
[4]   Bellomo R, Ronco C, Kellum JA, Mehta RL, Palevsky P. Acute renal
        failure - definition, outcome measures, animal models, fluid therapy and
        information technology needs: the Second International Consensus
        Conference of the Acute Dialysis Quality Initiative (ADQI) Group. *Crit
        Care* 2004;8:R204-12.
[5]   Clerico A, Galli C, Fortunato A, Ronco C. Neutrophil gelatinase-
        associated lipocalin (NGAL) as biomarker of acute kidney injury: a
        review of the laboratory characteristics and clinical evidences. *Clin
        Chem Lab Med* 2012;50:1505-17.
[6]   Cruz DN, Goh CY, Palazzuoli A, Slavin L, Calabrò A, Ronco C, Maisel
        A. Laboratory parameters of cardiac and kidney dysfunction in cardio-
        renal syndromes. *Heart Fail Rev* 2011;16:545-51.
[7]   Devarajan P. Review: neutrophil gelatinase-associated lipocalin: a
        troponin-like biomarker for human acute kidney injury. *Nephrology
        (Carlton)* 2010;15:419-28.
[8]   Bouman CS, Forni LG, Joannidis M. Biomarkers and acute kidney
        injury: dining with the Fisher King? *Intensive Care Med* 2010;36:381-4.
[9]   Devarajan P. Emerging biomarkers of acute kidney injury. *Contrib
        Nephrol* 2007;156:203-12.
[10]   Soni SS, Pophale R, Ronco C. New biomarkers for acute renal injury.
        Clin Chem Lab Med 2011;49:1257-63.
[11]   Thomas L and Huber AR. Renal function--estimation of glomerular
        filtration rate. *Clin Chem Lab Med* 2006;44:1295-302.
[12]   Heymsfield SB, Arteaga C, McManus C, Smith J, Moffitt S.
        Measurement of muscle mass in humans: validity of the 24-hour urinary
        creatinine method. *Am J Clin Nutr* 1983;37:478-94.
[13]   Perrone RD, Madias NE, Levey AS. Serum creatinine as an index of
        renal function: new insights into old concepts. *Clin Chem* 1992;38:1933-
        53.

[14] Shemesh O, Golbetz H, Kriss JP, Myers BD. Limitations of creatinine as a filtration marker in glomerulopathic patients. *Kidney Int* 1985;28:830-8.

[15] K/DOQI clinical practice guidelines for chronic kidney disease: evaluation, classification, and stratification. *Am J Kidney Dis* 2002; 39:S1-266.

[16] Spencer K. Analytical reviews in clinical biochemistry: the estimation of creatinine. *Ann Clin Biochem* 1986;23 (Pt 1):1-25.

[17] Miller BF and Winkler AW. The Renal Excretion of Endogenous Creatinine in Man. Comparison with Exogenous Creatinine and Inulin. *J Clin Invest* 1938;17:31-40.

[18] Cervellin G and di Somma S. Neutrophil gelatinase-associated lipocalin (NGAL): the clinician's perspective. *Clin Chem Lab Med* 2012;50:1489-93.

[19] Swain RR and Briggs SL. Positive interference with the Jaffe reaction by cephalosporin antibiotics. *Clin Chem* 1977;23:1340-2.

[20] Bowers LD. Kinetic serum creatinine assays I. The role of various factors in determining specificity. *Clin Chem* 1980;26:551-4.

[21] Myers GL, Miller WG, Coresh J, Fleming J, Greenberg N, Greene T, Hostetter T, Levey AS, Panteghini M, Welch M, Eckfeldt JH; National Kidney Disease Education Program Laboratory Working Group. Recommendations for improving serum creatinine measurement: a report from the Laboratory Working Group of the National Kidney Disease Education Program. *Clin Chem* 2006;52:5-18.

[22] Siekmann L. Determination of creatinine in human serum by isotope dilution-mass spectrometry. Definitive methods in clinical chemistry, IV. *J Clin Chem Clin Biochem* 1985;23:137-44.

[23] Carobene A, Ferrero C, Ceriotti F, Modenese A, Besozzi M, de Giorgi E, Franzin M, Franzini C, Kienle MG, Magni F. Creatinine measurement proficiency testing: assignment of matrix-adjusted ID GC-MS target values. *Clin Chem* 1997;43:1342-7.

[24] Lawson N, Lang T, Broughton A, Prinsloo P, Turner C, Marenah C. Creatinine assays: time for action? *Ann Clin Biochem* 2002;39:599-602.

[25] Levey AS, Bosch JP, Lewis JB, Greene T, Rogers N, Roth D. A more accurate method to estimate glomerular filtration rate from serum creatinine: a new prediction equation. Modification of Diet in Renal Disease Study Group. *Ann Intern Med* 1999;130:461-70.

[26] Rule AD, Larson TS, Bergstralh EJ, Slezak JM, Jacobsen SJ, Cosio FG. Using serum creatinine to estimate glomerular filtration rate: accuracy in

good health and in chronic kidney disease. *Ann Intern Med* 2004;141:929-37.

[27] Levey AS, Stevens LA, Schmid CH, Zhang YL, Castro AF 3rd, Feldman HI, Kusek JW, Eggers P, Van Lente F, Greene T, Coresh J; CKD-EPI (Chronic Kidney Disease Epidemiology Collaboration). A new equation to estimate glomerular filtration rate. *Ann Intern Med* 2009;150:604-12.

[28] Kidney Disease: Improving Global Outcomes (KDIGO) CKD Work Group. KDIGO 2012 clinical practice guideline for the evaluation and management of chronic kidney disease. *Kidney Int Supplements* 2013;3:1-150.

[29] Palevsky PM, Liu KD, Brophy PD, Chawla LS, Parikh CR, Thakar CV, Tolwani AJ, Waikar SS, Weisbord SD. KDOQI US commentary on the 2012 KDIGO clinical practice guideline for acute kidney injury. *Am J Kidney Dis* 2013;61:649-72.

[30] Kidney Disease: Improving Global Outcomes (KDIGO)Acute Kidney Injury Work Group. KDIGO Clinical Practice Guideline for Acute Kidney Injury. *Kidney Int Suppl* 2012;2:1-138.

[31] Mehta RL, Kellum JA, Shah SV, Molitoris BA, Ronco C, Warnock DG, Levin A; Acute Kidney Injury Network. Acute Kidney Injury Network: report of an initiative to improve outcomes in acute kidney injury. *Crit Care* 2007;11:R31.

[32] Levin A, Warnock DG, Mehta RL, Kellum JA, Shah SV, Molitoris BA, Ronco C; Acute Kidney Injury Network Working Group. Improving outcomes from acute kidney injury: report of an initiative. *Am J Kidney Dis* 2007;50:1-4.

[33] Mishra J, Dent C, Tarabishi R, Mitsnefes MM, Ma Q, Kelly C, Ruff SM, Zahedi K, Shao M, Bean J, Mori K, Barasch J, Devarajan P. Neutrophil gelatinase-associated lipocalin (NGAL) as a biomarker for acute renal injury after cardiac surgery. *Lancet* 2005;365:1231-8.

[34] Mishra J, Ma Q, Prada A, Mitsnefes M, Zahedi K, Yang J, Barasch J, Devarajan P. Identification of neutrophil gelatinase-associated lipocalin as a novel early urinary biomarker for ischemic renal injury. *J Am Soc Nephrol* 2003;14:2534-43.

[35] Flower DR, North AC, Sansom CE. The lipocalin protein family: structural and sequence overview. *Biochim Biophys Acta* 2000; 1482:9-24.

[36] Schmidt-Ott KM, Mori K, Li JY, Kalandadze A, Cohen DJ, Devarajan P, Barasch J. Dual action of neutrophil gelatinase-associated lipocalin. *J Am Soc Nephrol* 2007;18:407-13.

[37] Flo TH, Smith KD, Sato S, Rodriguez DJ, Holmes MA, Strong RK, Akira S, Aderem A. Lipocalin 2 mediates an innate immune response to bacterial infection by sequestrating iron. *Nature* 2004;432:917-21.

[38] Clifton MC, Corrent C, Strong RK. Siderocalins: siderophore-binding proteins of the innate immune system. *Biometals* 2009;22:557-64.

[39] Devarajan P. The promise of biomarkers for personalized renal cancer care. *Kidney Int* 2010;77:755-7.

[40] Devarajan P. Neutrophil gelatinase-associated lipocalin: new paths for an old shuttle. *Cancer Ther* 2007;5:463-70.

[41] Haase M, Bellomo R, Devarajan P, Schlattmann P, Haase-Fielitz A. Accuracy of neutrophil gelatinase-associated lipocalin (NGAL) in diagnosis and prognosis in acute kidney injury: a systematic review and meta-analysis. *Am J Kidney Dis* 2009;54:1012-24.

[42] Malyszko J, Bachorzewska-Gajewska H, Malyszko JS, Pawlak K, Dobrzycki S. Serum neutrophil gelatinase-associated lipocalin as a marker of renal function in hypertensive and normotensive patients with coronary artery disease. *Nephrology (Carlton)* 2008;13:153-6.

[43] Malyszko J, Malyszko JS, Bachorzewska-Gajewska H, Poniatowski B, Dobrzycki S, Mysliwiec M. Neutrophil gelatinase-associated lipocalin is a new and sensitive marker of kidney function in chronic kidney disease patients and renal allograft recipients. *Transplant Proc* 2009;41:158-61.

[44] Brunner HI, Mueller M, Rutherford C, Passo MH, Witte D, Grom A, Mishra J, Devarajan P. Urinary neutrophil gelatinase-associated lipocalin as a biomarker of nephritis in childhood-onset systemic lupus erythematosus. *Arthritis Rheum* 2006;54:2577-84.

[45] Ding H, He Y, Li K, Yang J, Li X, Lu R, Gao W. Urinary neutrophil gelatinase-associated lipocalin (NGAL) is an early biomarker for renal tubulointerstitial injury in IgA nephropathy. *Clin Immunol* 2007; 123:227-34.

[46] Yilmaz A, Sevketoglu E, Gedikbasi A, Karyagar S, Kiyak A, Mulazimoglu M, Aydogan G, Ozpacaci T, Hatipoglu S. Early prediction of urinary tract infection with urinary neutrophil gelatinase associated lipocalin. *Pediatr Nephrol* 2009;24:2387-92.

In: Neutrophil Gelatinase-Associated Lipocalin   ISBN: 978-1-63117-984-6
Editors: M. Hur and S. Di Somma   © 2014 Nova Science Publishers, Inc.

Chapter 12

Comparison of NGAL with other New Biomarkers for Kidney Disease

Francesco Vetrone, Benedetta De Berardinis
and Salvatore Di Somma[*]

Department of Medical-Surgery Sciences and
Translational Medicine, Sapienza University, Rome, Italy
Emergency medicine, Sant'Andrea Hospital, Rome, Italy

Abstract

Several studies and metaanalyses validated the utility of new kidney biomarkers, such as cystatina C (Cys C), kidney injury molecule-1 (KIM-1), interleukine- 18 (IL-18), N-acetyl-β-D-glucosamminidase (NAG), liver fatty-acid binding protein (L-FABP), and neutrophil gelatinase-associated lipocalin (NGAL).

Cys C is a marker of glomerular filtration because it is filtered by the glomerulus, reabsorbed completely, and is not secreted. Its urinary excretion is strictly linked to the severity of acute tubular damage and showed a good accuracy for the early diagnosis of AKI. KIM-1 is a type 1 transmembrane glycoprotein, which has an immunoglobulin and a mucin domain. The soluble form of human KIM-1 can be detected in the

[*] Correspondence: salvatore.disomma@uniroma1.it.

urine of patients with Acute Kidney Injury (AKI) and also in patients with focal glomerulo-sclerosis, IgA nephropathy, or membrano-proliferative glomerulonephritis, identifying chronic tubulointerstitial damage.

IL-18, a member of the IL-1 cytokine superfamily and known as an interferon-γ-inducing factor, regulates innate and adaptive immunity. It is an important mediator of acute ischemic AKI. NAG, a lysosomal brush border enzyme of the proximal tubule cells, is released into the urine after renal injury. This chapter provides an overview on each kidney biomarker in comparison with NGAL.

Introduction

Although technical innovations for the treatment of acute renal damage, including renal replacement therapy (RRT), have been developed, AKI is still associated with a high mortality in the critically ill patients [1]. For the early diagnosis of AKI in acute disease, current assessment of renal function is based on serum creatinine level (sCr) and blood urea nitrogen (BUN).

Unfortunately, these two biomarkers have, in this setting, poor sensitivity and specificity for early detection of acute damage in kidney function; as a consequence new biomarkers are needed.

Compared to sCr, these new biomarkers should be more precise, sensitive, and specific in order to reduce time of AKI diagnosis, monitor kidney functions, and provide information for patients risk stratification and prognosis. There are several emerging biomarkers for early diagnosis and prognosis of AKI, and a physician can hardly decide the more suitable and efficient one, in order to start promptly an adequate treatment as consequence of a fast and adequate AKI diagnosis.

Cys C, KIM-1, IL-18, L-FABP, NAG, and NGAL are the mostly used ones. The use of these biomarkers of acute kidney damage could be of great utility in order to distinguish AKI from volume responsive renal dysfunction, chronic kidney disease (CKD), or normal renal function [2-4].

Furthermore, these biomarkers could contribute to the diagnosis of AKI by identifying a subgroup with "subclinical AKI" where there may be injury even in the absence of sCr increase [5, 6], thus leading to an earlier risk stratifica-tion of patients with prompt and specific treatment strategies [7].

Comparison of NGAL with Other Biomarkers for Kidney Diseases

Creatinine (sCr)

Creatinine (sCr) is the standard serum biomarker to detect AKI. It is cheap, non-invasive, fast, and can be used to establish the glomerular filtration rate (GFR), but it demonstrated several limitations in clinical practice. sCr level can change with patient's age, gender, muscle mass, body nutrition, body weight, hydration status, and medications.

Moreover, at low GFR, the sCr levels results in an overestimation of renal function. Finally, in AKI, sCr does not reflect accurately kidney function, until steady-state equilibrium has been reached [8].

This need for repeated sCr evaluations and monitoring of urinary output for several days after admission could therefore result in a delay in appropriate therapy [9-12].

The application of the Risk, Injury, Failure; Loss, End-Stage Renal Disease (RIFLE) criteria to patients presenting to emergency department (ED) is quite challenging, since decrease in urine output is not quantified, and a pre-hospital stable baseline sCr is, in most patients, not available. Nickolas et al. [2, 3] using a single urine NGAL measurement in the ED demonstrated that this biomarker is superior to sCr in detecting AKI, and has a significant prognostic ability for these patients.

Furthermore, our group using blood NGAL with a point-of-care system recently showed that, compared to sCr, NGAL was significantly better in early detecting renal dysfunction in patients hospitalized for different acute diseases (Figure 1) [7].

Blood Urea Nitrogen (BUN)

Blood urea nitrogen (BUN) is commonly used for detecting acute renal damage, although it is not a specific marker of AKI. BUN is affected by many renal and non-renal factors that are independent of kidney injury or kidney function, such as high-protein diet, hemorrhage, trauma, and glucocorticoid therapy [13].

A   B

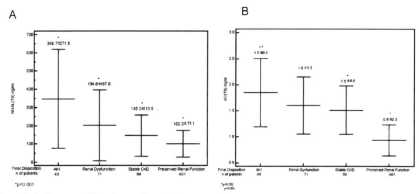

Figure 1. Mean ± SD neutrophil gelatinase-associated lipocalin (NGAL) (A) and serum creatinine (sCr) (B) at T0 by final diagnosis.

Cystatina C (Cys C)

Cystatin C (Cys C) is a cysteine protease inhibitor synthesized by all nucleated cells in the body. It is a marker of glomerular filtration, since it is filtered by the glomerulus, completely reabsorbed by tubular cells, and is not secreted in the urine [14]. Furthermore, CysC urinary excretion is strictly linked to the severity of acute tubular damage and shows a good accuracy for the early diagnosis of AKI [15]. As shown by Herget-Rosenthal et al. [15] Cys C was a useful marker of AKI and was able to detect AKI one to two days earlier compared with sCr. Similar results were found by Ahlström, et al. [16]. In a small study on non-diabetics patients with normal sCr undergoing elective PCI, Cys C showed a significant rise at 8 and 24 hours after the procedure, while NGAL showed a significant rise after 4, 8, and 24 hours after PCI, allowing a much earlier identification of contrast-induced nephropathy (CIN) [17]. A similar result was found in another study showing more power of NGAL compared with Cys C in identifying CIN [18].

Finally, in diagnosis of AKI in CIN, Liu et al. [19] described that NGAL has a sensitivity and specificity of 87% and 80%, while Cys C had 76% of sensitivity and 81% of specificity. In the same study, plasma NGAL level peaked at 4 hours after PCI, while Cys C level peaked only after 24 hours [19].

NGAL and Cys C were also studied in the diagnosis of Type1 cardio-renal syndrome (CRS). Alvelos et al. [20] studied patients admitted with acute heart failure (AHF) and demonstrated that, 30% of them developed type 1 CRS within 72 hours.

The area under the receiver operating characteristics (ROC) curve (AUC) for AKI in these patients for NGAL was 0.93 (CI 0.88 - 0.98) with a best cut-off value of 170 ng/mL with a sensitivity of 100% and a specificity of 86.7%; while the AUC of CysC was significantly lower: 0.68 (0.54 - 0.82). Haase et al. [21] tried to correlate plasma level of NGAL and serum Cys C in 100 adults with the duration, severity, and length of stay in intensive care units (ICU).

The AUC for AKI prediction was 0.77 (CI 0.63 - 0.91) for NGAL and 0.76 (CI 0.61 - 0.91) for Cys C. In this study, NGAL and Cys C were both independent predictors for the severity of AKI and duration of ICU stay after adult cardiac surgery. In critically ill septic patient, Aydogdu et al. [22] demonstrated that plasma, urinary Cys C and urinary NGAL were useful markers in predicting AKI.

Kidney Injury Molecule-1 (KIM-1)

Kidney injury molecule-1 (KIM-1) is a type 1 transmembrane glycoprotein, which has an immunoglobulin and a mucin domain. Structure and expression data suggest that KIM-1 is an epithelial cell adhesion molecule up-regulated in the cells, which are dedifferentiated and undergoing replication. In healthy kidney, KIM-1 is undetectable, but is overexpressed in the apical membrane of proximal tubule epithelial cells after ischemic or nephrotoxic injury [23]. Furthermore, KIM-1 is believed to participate in the regeneration process after epithelial injury [24]. KIM-1 is absent in the glomerulus, peritubular interstitial cells, or inner medullary cells. The soluble form of human KIM-1 can be detected in the urine of patients with AKI but also in the patients with focal glomerulosclerosis, IgA nephropathy, or membranoprolife-rative glomerulonephritis, identifying chronic tubulointerstitial damage [25, 26].

Urine KIM-1, in combination with uNGAL and other kidney injury biomarkers, is able to predict AKI 3 hours after cardiac surgery with an AUC of 0.75 and 0.78, respectively [27].

In a large study on paediatric patients who underwent cardiopulmonary bypass (CPB), Krawczesky et al. [28] demonstrated that urine NGAL was significantly increased in AKI patients 2 hours and 6 hours after surgery while urine KIM-1 12 hours after operation; NGAL still had the highest discrimination power ($P < 0.0001$). Wasilewska et al. [29] in children with severe congenital hydronephrosis compared urine NGAL and KIM-1 in detecting kidney injury.

They concluded that both biomarkers were able to detect worsening of urinary tract obstruction but not progression of chronic kidney disease. On the contrary, the study by de Geus et al. [30] showed early expression levels of NGAL and KIM-1 prior to AKI diagnosis.

The rise in KIM-1 overtime even when AKI does not develop may be explained by the ability of this biomarker to detect subclinical injury, because KIM-1 is a transmembrane glycoprotein exclusively present in the epithelial cells that survives after injury [25, 31].

These results were also found by Liangos et al. [32]. They found that KIM-1 has a higher sensitivity and specificity for AKI diagnosis (92% and 58%, respectively), compared with NGAL (sensitivity 67% and specificity 11%), 2 hours following CPB. Jugbauer et al. [33] also demonstrated that KIM-1 and NGAL are able to indicate renal tubular involvement in chronic heart failure patients, and could therefore be considered potentially biomarkers of the CRS, providing additional prognostic information on heart failure.

Interleukin 18 (IL-18)

IL-18, a member of the IL-1 cytokine superfamily and known as an interferon-γ-inducing factor, regulates innate and adaptive immunity [34]. IL-18 is synthesized in an inactive form by several tissues including monocytes, macrophages, and proximal tubular epithelial cells. This interleukin binds IL-18r complex expressed on hematopoietic cells, endothelial cells, and smooth muscle cells.

Following AKI, IL-18 levels in the kidneys double, and several animal studies demonstrated an elevation of IL-18 following hypoxia or ischemic AKI [35].

In patients with acute respiratory distress syndrome in ICU, urine IL-18 (uIL-18) > 100 pg/mL were associated with an increased risk of AKI of 6.5 and predicted mortality [36]. Ling et al. [37] demonstrated that uNGAL and uIL-18 were similar biomarkers in detecting AKI earlier than sCr.

Siew et al. [38], in a prospective study of adult ICU population, evaluated the ability of uIL-18 to predict AKI, death, and RRT. In patients who developed AKI, the predictive value of IL-18 showed an AUC of 0.62 (CI 0.54 − 0.69); moreover, in patients with sepsis, its urine levels were constantly higher and independently predictive of poor clinical outcome.

Liver Fatty-Acid Binding Protein (L-FABP)

In 1992, Maatman et al. [39, 40] discovered the presence of two variants of fatty-acid binding protein (FABP) in the kidney: H-FABP and L-FABP. Liver FABP (L-FABP) is a 15 kDA protein that belongs to the superfamily of the FABP. L-FABP is not only expressed in the liver, but also in the intestine, pancreas, kidneys, lungs, and stomach. Urinary L-FABP is undetectable in healthy subjects. Under ischemic condition, the proximal tubular reabsorption of L-FABP is reduced, and it can be measured in the urine by enzyme-linked immunosorbent assay [41, 28].

Zeng et al. [42] evaluated the power of NGAL and L-FABP to detect the occurrence of AKI and to predict the recovery from renal dysfunction in major surgery patients. In 37 patients that developed AKI, the peak levels of NGAL and L-FABP occurred 12 and 4 hours postoperatively (16.4- and 172.0-fold compared to baseline), respectively. The most predictive model on ROC curve was obtained with NGAL at 12 hours.

N – Acetyl- β- D- Glucosamminidase (NAG)

NAG, a lysosomal brush border enzyme of the proximal tubule cells, is released into the urine after renal injury. KIM-1 is elevated in symptomatic heart failure patients as pointed out in a study where KIM-1, NAG, and NGAL were assessed in unstable chronic patients [33]. In patients with systolic heart failure, Damman et al. [43] showed that NAG works as biomarker of tubular injury and could mirror renal injury due to venous congestion.

They demonstrated that while urinary KIM-1 and NAG rapidly increased after diuretic withdrawal (with parallel BNP increase), urinary NGAL was not affected. Moreover, both urinary biomarkers returned to baseline values after reintroduction of diuretic.

Conclusion

Several studies and meta-analysis validated the utility of the assessment of new biomarkers such as: Cys C, KIM-1, NAG, IL-18, L-FABP, and NGAL for AKI diagnosis. The level of these biomarkers has been correlated with the severity (stage) of AKI and assessed for their predictive value for RRT, mortality, or renal functional recovery. Furthermore, all these biomarkers could identify the presence of subclinical damage in the kidney with preserved function, allowing establishing the use of kidney injury biomarkers in the early detection of renal involvement and risk stratification of patients.

Comparing the results between AKI biomarkers among several studies in different populations, NGAL seems to have the highest evidences for diagnostic and prognostic values of acute renal damage.

References

[1]   Brar SS, Hiremath S, Dangas G, Mehran R, Brar SK, Leon MB. Sodium bicarbonate for the prevention of contrast induced-acute kidney injury: a systematic review and meta-analysis. *Clin. J. Am. Soc. Nephrol.* 2009;4:1584-92.

[2]   Nickolas TL, Schmidt-Ott KM, Canetta P, Forster C, Singer E, Sise M, Elger A, Maarouf O, Sola-Del Valle DA, O'Rourke M, Sherman E, Lee P, Geara A, Imus P, Guddati A, Polland A, Rahman W, Elitok S, Malik N, Giglio J, El-Sayegh S, Devarajan P, Hebbar S, Saggi SJ, Hahn B, Kettritz R, Luft FC, Barasch J. Diagnostic and prognostic stratification in the emergency department using urinary biomarkers of nephron damage a multicenter prospective cohort study. *J. Am. Coll. Cardiol.* 2012;59:246-55.

[3]   Nickolas TL, O'Rourke MJ, YangJ, Sise ME, Canetta PA, Barasch N, Buchen C, Khan F, Mori K, Giglio J, Devarajan P, Barasch J. Sensitivity and specificity of a single emergency department measurement of urinary neutrophil gelatinase–associated lipocalin for diagnosing acute kidney injury. *Ann. Inter. Med.* 2008;148:810-9.

[4]   Urbschat A, Obermüller N, Haferkamp A. Biomarkers of kidney injury. *Biomarkers* 2011;16 Suppl. 1: S22-30.

[5]   Ronco C, Kellum JA, Haase M. Subclinical AKI is still AKI. *Crit. Care* 2012;16:313.

[6]   Haase M, Devarajan P, Haase-Fielitz A, Bellomo R, Cruz DN, Wagener, G, Krawczeski CD, Koyner JL, Murray P, Zappitelli M, Goldstein SL, Makris K, Ronco C, Martensson J, Martling CR, Venge P, Siew E, Ware LB, Ikizler TA, Mertens PR. The outcome of neutrophil gelatinase-associated lipocalin positive sub-clinical acute kidney injury. *J. Am. Coll. Cardiol.* 2011;57:1752-61.

[7]   Di Somma S, Magrini L, De Berardinis B, Marino R, Ferri E, Moscatelli P, Ballarino P, Carpinteri G, Noto P, Gliozzo B, Paladino L, Di Stasio E.

Additive value of blood neutrophil gelatinase-associated lipocalin to clinical judgement in acute kidney injury diagno-sis and mortality prediction in patients hospitalized from the emergency department. *Crit. Care* 2013;17(1):R29.

[8] Nguyen MT, Devarajan P. Biomarkers for the early detection of acute kidney injury. *Pediatr. Nephrol.* 2008;23:2151-7.

[9] Joslin J, Ostermann M. Care of the critically ill emergency department patient with acute kidney injury. *Emerg. Med. Int.* 2012;2012:760623.

[10] Bellomo R, Ronco C, Kellum JA, Mehta RL, Palevsky P. Acute renal failure, definition, outcome measures, animal models fluid therapy and information technology needs: the Second International Consensus Conference of the Acute Dialysis Quality Initiative (ADQI) Group. *Crit. Care* 2004;8: R204-12.

[11] Mehta RL, Kellum JA, Shah SV, Molitoris BA, Ronco C, Warnock D. G, Levin A. Acute Kidney Injury Network. Acute Kidney Injury Network: report of an initiative to improve outcomes in acute kidney injury. *Crit. Care* 2007;11:R31.

[12] Kidney Disease: Improving Global Outcomes (KDIGO) Acute Kidney Injury Work Group. KDIGO Clinical Practice Guideline for Acute Kidney Injury. *Kidney Inter.* Suppl. 2012;2:1–138.

[13] Proulx NL, Akbari A, Garg AX, Rostom A, Jaffey J, Clark HD. Measured creatinine clearance from timed urine collections substan-tially overestimates glomerular filtration rate in patients with liver cirrhosis: a systematic review and individual patient meta-analysis. *Nephrol. Dial. Transplant.* 2005;20:1617-22.

[14] Dharnidharka VR, Kwon C, Stevens G. Serum cystatin C is superior to serum creatinine as a marker of kidney function: a meta-analysis. *Am. J. Kidney Dis.* 2002;40:221-6.

[15] Herget-Rosenthal S, Marggraf G, Hüsing J, Göring F, Pietruck F, Janssen O, Philipp T, Kribben A. Early detection of acute renal failure by serum cystatin C. *Kidney Int.* 2004;66:1115-22.

[16] Ahlström A, Tallgren M, Peltonen S, Pettilä V. Evolution and predictive power of serum cystatin C in acute renal failure. *Clin. Nephrol.* 2004;62:344-50.

[17] Bachorzewska-Gajewska H, Malyszko J, Sitniewska E, Malyszko JS, Poniatowski B, Pawlak K, Dobrzycki S. NGAL (neutrophil gelati-nase-associated lipocalin) and cystatin C: are they good predictors of contrast nephropathy after percutaneous coronary interventions in patients with

stable angina and normal serum creatinine? *Int. J. Cardiol.* 2008;127:290-1.

[18] Bachorzewska-Gajewska H, Malyszko J, Sitniewska E, Malyszko JS, Pawlak K, Mysliwiec M, Lawnicki S, Szmitkowski M, Dobrzycki S. Could neutrophil-gelatinase-associated lipocalin and cystatin C predict the development of contrast-induced nephropathy after percutaneous coronary interventions in patients with stable angina and normal serum creatinine values? *Kidney Blood Press Res.* 2007;30:408-15.

[19] Liu XL, Wang ZJ, Yang Q, Yu M, Shen H, Nie B, Han HY, Gao F, Zhou YJ. Plasma neutrophil-gelatinase-associated lipocalin and cystatin C could early diagnose contrast-induced acute kidney injury in patients with renal insufficiency undergoing an elective percutaneous coronary intervention. *Chin. Med. J.* (Engl.) 2012;125:1051-6.

[20] Alvelos M, Pimentel R, Pinho E, Gomes A, Lourenço P, Teles MJ, Almeida P, Guimarães JT, Bettencourt P. Neutrophil gelatinase-associated lipocalin in the diagnosis of type 1 cardio-renal syndrome in the general ward. *Clin. J. Am. Soc. Nephrol.* 2011;6:476-81.

[21] Haase M, Bellomo R, Devarajan P, Ma Q, Bennett MR, Möckel M, Matalanis G, Dragun D, Haase-Fielitz A. Novel biomarkers early predict the severity of acute kidney injury after cardiac surgery in adults. *Ann. Thorac. Surg.* 2009;88:124-30.

[22] Aydoğdu M, Gürsel G, Sancak B, Yeni S, Sarı G, Taşyürek S, Türk M, Yüksel S, Senes M, Ozis TN. The use of plasma and urine neutrophil gelatinase associated lipocalin (NGAL) and cystatin C in early diagnosis of septic acute kidney injury in critically ill patients. *Dis. Markers* 2013;34:237-46.

[23] Ichimura T, Bonventre JV, Bailly V, Wei H, Hession CA, Cate RL, Sanicola M. Kidney injury molecule-1 (KIM-1), a putative epithelial cell adhesion molecule containing a novel immunoglobulin domain, is up-regulated in renal cells after injury. *J. Biol. Chem.* 1998; 273:4135-42.

[24] Ichimura T, Asseldonk EJ, Humphreys BD, Gunaratnam L, Duffield JS, Bonventre JV. Kidney injury molecule-1 is a phosphati-dylserine receptor that confers a phagocytic phenotype on epithelial cells. *J. Clin. Invest.* 2008;118:1657-68.

[25] Han WK, Bailly V, Abichandani R, Thadhani R, Bonventre JV. Kidney Injury Molecule-1 (KIM-1): a novel biomarker for human renal proximal tubule injury. *Kidney Int.* 2002;62:237-44.

[26] Van Timmeren MM, van den Heuvel MC, Bailly V, Bakker SJ, van Goor H, Stegeman CA. Tubular kidney injury molecule-1 (KIM-1) in human renal disease. *J. Pathol.* 2007;212:209-17.

[27] Han WK, Wagener G, Zhu Y, Wang S, Lee HT. Urinary bio-markers in the early detection of acute kidney injury after cardiac surgery. *Clin. J. Am. Soc. Nephrol.* 2009;4:873-82.

[28] Krawczeski CD, Goldstein SL, Woo JG, Wang Y, Piyaphanee N, Ma Q, Bennett M, Devarajan P. Temporal relationship and predictive value of urinary acute kidney injury biomarkers after pediatric cardiopulmonary bypass. *J. Am. Coll. Cardiol.* 2011;58:2301-9.

[29] Wasilewska A, Taranta-Janusz K, Dębek W, Zoch-Zwierz W, Kuroczycka-Saniutycz E. KIM-1 and NGAL: new markers of obstructive nephropathy. *Pediatr. Nephrol.* 2011;26:579-86.

[30] De Geus HR, Fortrie G, Betjes MG, van Schaik RH, Groeneveld AJ. Time of injury affects urinary biomarker predictive values for acute kidney injury in critically ill, non-septic patients. *BMC Nephrol.* 2013;14:273.

[31] Koyner JL, Vaidya VS, Bennett MR, Ma Q, Worcester E, Akhter SA, Raman J, Jeevanandam V, O'Connor MF, Devarajan P, Bonventre JV, Murray PT. Urinary biomarkers in the clinical prognosis and early detection of acute kidney injury. *Clin. J. Am. Soc. Nephrol.* 2010;5:2154-65.

[32] Liangos O, Tighiouart H, Perianayagam MC, Kolyada A, Han WK, Wald R, Bonventre JV, Jaber BL. Comparative analysis of urinary biomarkers for early detection of acute kidney injury following cardiopulmonary bypass. *Biomarkers* 2009;14:423-31.

[33] Jungbauer CG, Birner C, Jung B, Buchner S, Lubnow M, von Bary C, Endemann D, Banas B, Mack M, Böger CA, Riegger G, Luchner A. Kidney injury molecule-1 and N-acetyl-β-D-glucosami-nidase in chronic heart failure: possible biomarkers of cardiorenal syndrome. *Eur. J. Heart Fail.* 2011;13:1104-10.

[34] Gracie JA, Robertson SE, McInnes IB. Interleukin-18. *J. Leukoc. Biol.* 2003;73:213-24.

[35] He Z, Dursun B, Oh DJ, Lu L, Faubel S, Edelstein CL. Macro-phages are not the source of injurious interleukin-18 in ischemic acute kidney injury in mice. *Am. J. Physiol. Renal Physiol.* 2009;296:F535-42.

[36] Parikh CR, Abraham E, Ancukiewicz M, Edelstein CL. Urine IL-18 is an early diagnostic marker for acute kidney injury and predicts mortality in the intensive care unit. *J. Am. Soc. Nephrol.* 2005;16:3046-52.

[37] Ling W, Zhaohui N, Ben H, Leyi G, Jianping L, Huili D, Jiaqi Q. Urinary IL-18 and NGAL as early predictive biomarkers in contrast-induced nephropathy after coronary angiography. *Nephron. Clin. Pract.* 2008;108:c176-81.

[38] Siew ED, Ikizler TA, Gebretsadik T, Shintani A, Wickersham N, Bossert F, Peterson JF, Parikh CR, May AK, Ware, LB. Elevated urinary IL-18 levels at the time of ICU admission predict adverse clinical outcomes. *Clin. J. Am. Soc. Nephrol.* 2010;5:1497-505.

[39] Maatman RG, Van Kuppevelt TH, Veerkamp JH. Two types of fatty acid-binding protein in human kidney. Isolation, characterization and localization. *Biochem. J.* 1991;273:759-66.

[40] Maatman RG, van de Westerlo EM, van Kuppevelt TH, Veer-kamp J. H. Molecular identification of the liver- and the heart-type fatty acid-binding proteins in human and rat kidney. Use of the reverse trans-criptase polymerase chain reaction. *Biochem. J.* 1992;288:285-90.

[41] Yamamoto T, Noiri E, Ono Y, Doi K, Negishi K, Kamijo A, Kimura K, Fujita T, Kinukawa T, Taniguchi H, Nakamura K, Goto M, Shinozaki N, Ohshima S, Sugaya T. Renal L-type fatty acid--binding protein in acute ischemic injury. *J. Am. Soc. Nephrol.* 2007;18:2894-902.

[42] Zeng XF, Li JM, Tan Y, Wang ZF, He Y, Chang J, Zhang H, Zhao H, Bai X, Xie F, Sun J, Zhang Y. Performance of urinary NGAL and L-FABP in predicting acute kidney injury and subsequent renal recovery: a cohort study based on major surgeries. *Clin. Chem. Lab. Med.* 2013 Nov. 29:1-8. doi: 10.1515/cclm-2013-0823. [Epub. ahead of print].

[43] Damman K, Ng Kam Chuen MJ, MacFadyen RJ, Lip GYH, Gaze D, Collinson PO, Hillege HL, van Oeveren W, Voors AA, van Veldhuisen DJ. Volume status and diuretic therapy in systolic heart failure and the detection of early abnormalities in renal and tubular function. *J. Am. Coll. Cardiol.* 2011;57:2233-41.

In: Neutrophil Gelatinase-Associated Lipocalin   ISBN: 978-1-63117-984-6
Editors: M. Hur and S. Di Somma   © 2014 Nova Science Publishers, Inc.

Chapter 13

NGAL: A Marker for Acute Kidney Injury

W. Frank Peacock, M.D., FACEP*

Emergency Medicine, Baylor College of Medicine,
Ben Taub General Hospital, Houston, Texas, US

Abstract

Neutrophil gelatinase-associated lipocalin (NGAL), a member of the lipocalin family of proteins and secreted by kidney tubule cells at low levels, increases dramatically after ischemic, septic, or nephrotoxic renal injury.

Identifying acute kidney injury (AKI) early in its course could allow interventions preventing worsening renal function (WRF), thus the use of NGAL to detect early AKI may be of considerable clinical importance. The use of NGAL as a marker of AKI has been specifically evaluated in the emergency department (ED), a population with uncharacterized illness and whose kidney injury is often evolving.

Data in literature demonstrated that the assessment of patient's initial blood NGAL when admitted to hospital from ED improved the initial clinical diagnosis of AKI, moreover NGAL assessment coupled with the ED physician's clinical judgment may prove useful in deciding the appropriate strategies for patients at risk for the development of AKI.

* Correspondence: W. Frank Peacock. E-mail: Frankpeacock@gmail.com.

Finally, presentation NGAL > 400 ng/mL had the highest predictive value for in-hospital patient's mortality of all the evaluated predictive parameters.

Introduction

Neutrophil gelatinase-associated lipocalin (NGAL), a member of the lipocalin family of proteins and secreted by kidney tubule cells at low levels, increases dramatically after ischemic, septic, or nephrotoxic renal injury [1-3]. Because no test detects acute kidney injury (AKI) at the time of onset, the diagnosis of worsening renal function (WRF) is achieved by serial creatinine measurements. Unfortunately, creatinine is an insensitive and late AKI marker [4]. Identifying AKI early in its course could allow interventions preventing WRF, thus the use of NGAL to detect early AKI may be of considerable clinical importance.

Increased NGAL, occurs in as little as 2 hours after renal injury, precedes creatinine increase by 12 to 24 hours [5], and is highly predictive of the subsequent development of AKI. Although sometimes reversible, AKI is associated with increased morbidity, prolonged hospital stay, the need for dialysis, and potential mortality. A recent review reported on 203 clinical trials from a wide range of pathology, 56 of which identified NGAL as an early AKI biomarker [6].

The use of NGAL as a marker of AKI has been specifically evaluated in the emergency department (ED), a population with uncharacterized illness and whose kidney injury is often evolving. In one prospective consecutive enrollment study of 635 patients presenting to the ED, NGAL more accurately differentiated AKI from pre-renal azotemia, CKD, and those with normal renal function vs. creatinine and other renal injury markers [7]. ED differentiation of renal risk using NGAL could allow renal protection strategies to be initiated earlier than when creatinine is used for diagnosis. In a second study using a point-of-care ED NGAL assay in 661 potentially septic patients, NGAL was considerably more sensitive than serial creatinine for the identification of subsequent renal failure or death [8].

Other studies support that early NGAL measurement may be useful at ED presentation to identify patients at risk of AKI. Bagshaw et al. [9] measured NGAL at 0, 12, 24, and 48 hours in 83 septic patients, finding that there were significantly higher NGAL levels at enrollment in patients with septic AKI.

Finally, a recent prospective multicenter Italian study of 665 hospitalized patients demonstrated the additive value of NGAL to clinical decision making (Figure 1.) [10].

In this study, serial NGAL and creatinine were measured during the first 72 hours, and the ED physician indicated their initial assessment of the probability of AKI. Defined by RIFLE AKI criteria adjudicated by nephrologists after study completion, AKI occurred in 49 (7%) of patients, however, the assessment of AKI by the ED was that it was present in 218 (33%).

While the ED physician's initial judgement was inaccurate, overpredicting the diagnosis of AKI in 27% and missing the diagnosis of AKI in 20%, NGAL was much more precise. The area under the receiver operating characteristic curve (AUC) for NGAL predicting AKI at presentation was 0.80.

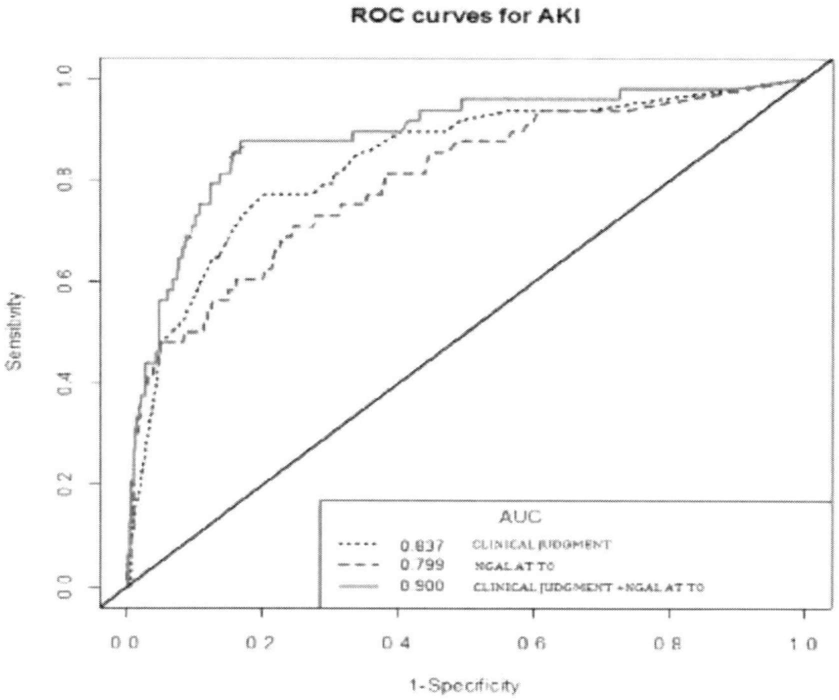

ROC curves for AKI

AUC		
0.837	CLINICAL JUDGMENT	
0.799	NGAL AT T0	
0.900	CLINICAL JUDGMENT + NGAL AT T0	

Figure 1. T0 receiver-operatingcharacteristic (ROC) curves by adjudicated acute kidney injury (AKI) based on neutrophilgelatinase-associatedlipocalin (NGAL), clinical judgment of developing AKI, and NGAL combined with clinical judgement [10].

Further, when presentation NGAL was added to the ED physician's initial clinical judgment, the overall accuracy improved (AUC for predicting AKI equaled 0.90). This was significantly better than the presentation estimated glomerular filtration rate (eGFR) calculated by either the modification of diet in renal disease (MDRD) equation (0.78) or Cockroft-Gault formula (0.78) (P = 0.022 and P = 0.020, respectively).

Finally, the clinical impact at presentation of the combination of NGAL and clinical judgment vs. creatinine, resulted in a net reclassification index of 32.4%. Further, serial NGAL at presentation and 6 hours later provided a negative predictive value of 98% for ruling out diagnosis. Finally, presentation NGAL > 400 ng/mL had the highest predictive value for in-hospital patient's mortality of all the evaluated predictive parameters.

Because of the steep increase in contrast studies performed in contemporary emergency medicine practice, another potential application for the use of NGAL includes that of identifying patients at risk for, or subsequently sustaining, contrast-induced nephropathy (CIN).

CIN can be defined as a creatinine increase of 25% to 50% above baseline, and general occurs within 24 hours after contrast exposure. CIN is the third leading cause of nosocomial AKI and has an incidence from 0 to 50%, depending on the absence or presence of risk factors [11].

While roughly 50% of CIN occurs after cardiac angiography, about one-third of cases follow exposure to computed tomography [12].

In one study of 60 non-diabetics with an initially normal creatinine and undergoing elective percutaneous coronary intervention (PCI), NGAL demonstrated a good sensitivity and specificity for CIN [13]. In cases of CIN, NGAL increased 2, 4, and 8 hours after PCI, occurring much earlier than increases in either creatinine or cystatin C. In another study of 100 patients undergoing PCI, 11% developed CIN [14]. Similar to the first trial, NGAL was significantly higher within 2 hours of PCI. This was compared to cystatin C, which did not rise until 8 and 24 hours after PCI in the CIN cohort.

Conclusion

These trials support the fact that NGAL is a sensitive and early biomarker of AKI after contrast exposure and suggest NGAL is an effective early biomarker for identifying AKI after CIN.

Disclosures: Research Grants: Abbott, Alere, Cardiorentis, Roche, The Medicine's Company, Thermo-Fisher; Consultant: Abbott, Alere, BG Medicine, Cardiorentis, Jannsen, Lily, The Medicine's Company, Singulex; Ownership Interest: Comprehensive Research Associates LLC, Emergencies in Medicine LLC.

References

[1]   Mishra, J., Mori, K., Ma, Q., Kelly, C., Barasch, J., Devarajan, P. Neutrophil gelatinase-associated lipocalin: a novel early urinary bio-marker for cisplatin nephrotoxicity. *Am J Nephrol* 2004;24:307–15.

[2]   Mori, K., Nakao, K. Neutrophil gelatinase-associated lipocalin as the real-time indicator of active kidney damage. *Kidney Int* 2007;71:967–70.

[3]   Hirsch, R., Dent, C., Pfriem, H., Allen, J., Beekman, R. H. 3rd, Ma, Q., Dastrala, S., Bennett, M., Mitsnefes, M., Devarajan, P. NGAL is an early predictive biomarker of contrast-induced nephropathy in children. *Pediatr Nephrol* 2007;22:2089–95.

[4]   Devarajan, P. Emerging biomarkers of acute kidney injury. *Contrib Nephrol* 2007;156:203–12.

[5]   Mishra, J., Dent, C., Tarabishi, R., Mitsnefes, M. M., Ma, Q., Kelly, C., Ruff, S. M., Zahedi, K., Shao, M., Bean, J., Mori, K., Barasch, J., Devarajan, P. Neutrophil gelatinase-associated lipocalin (NGAL) as a biomarker for acute renal injury after cardiac surgery. *Lancet* 2005;365: 1231–8.

[6]   Peacock, W. F., Maisel, A., Kim, J., Ronco, C. Neutrophil gelatinase associated lipocalin in acute kidney injury. *Postgrad. Med* 2013;125: 82-93.

[7]   Nickolas, T. L., O'Rourke, M. J., Yang, J., Sise, M. E., Canetta, P. A., Barasch, N., Buchen, C., Khan, F., Mori, K., Giglio, J., Devarajan, P., Barasch, J. Sensitivity and specificity of a single emergency department measurement of urinary neutrophil gelatinase-associated lipocalin for diagnosing acute kidney injury. *Ann Intern Med* 2008;148:810–9.

[8]   Shapiro, N. I., Trzeciak, S., Hollander, J. E., Birkhahn, R., Otero, R., Osborn, T. M., Moretti, E., Nguyen, H. B., Gunnerson, K., Milzman, D., Gaieski, D. F., Goyal, M., Cairns, C. B., Kupfer, K., Lee, S. W., Rivers, E. P. The diagnostic accuracy of plasma neutrophil gelatinase-associated lipocalin in the prediction of acute kidney injury in emergency depart-ment patients with suspected sepsis. *Ann Emerg Med* 2010;56:52–9, e1.

[9]   Bagshaw, S. M., Bennett, M., Haase, M., Haase-Fielitz, A., Egi, M., Morimatsu, H., D'amico, G., Goldsmith, D., Devarajan, P., Bellomo, R. Plasma and urine neutrophil gelatinase-associated lipocalin in septic versus non-septic acute kidney injury in critical illness. *Inten. Care Med.* 2010;36:452–61.

[10] Disomma, S., Magrini, L., De Berardinis, B., Marino, R., Ferri, E., Moscatelli, P., Ballarino, P., Carpinteri, G., Noto, P., Gliozzo, B., Paladino, L., Di Stasio, E. Additive value of blood neutrophil gelatinase associated lipocalin to clinical judgement in acute kidney injury diagnosis and mortality prediction in patients hospitalized from the emergency department. *Crit Care* 2013;17:R29.

[11] Nash, K., Hafeez, A., Hou, S. Hospital-acquired renal insufficiency. *Am J Kidney Dis* 2002;39:930–6.

[12] Marenzi, G., Lauri, G., Assanelli, E., Campodonico, J., De Metrio, M., Marana, I., Grazi, M., Veglia, F., Bartorelli, A. L. Contrast-induced nephropathy in patients undergoing primary angioplasty for acute myocardial infarction. *J Am Col. Cardiol* 2004;44:1780–5.

[13] Bachorzewska-Gajewska, H., Malyszko, J., Sitniewska, E., Malyszko, J. S., Poniatowski, B., Pawlak, K., Dobrzycki, S. NGAL (neutrophil gelatinase-associated lipocalin) and cystatin C: are they good predictors of contrast nephropathy after percutaneous coronary interventions in patients with stable angina and normal serum creatinine? *Int. J Cardiol* 2008;127:290–1.

[14] Bachorzewska-Gajewska, H., Malyszko, J., Sitniewska, E., Malyszko, J. S., Pawlak, K., Mysliwiec, M., Lawnicki, S., Szmitkowski, M., Dobrzycki, S. Could neutrophil-gelatinase-associated lipocalin and cystatin C predict the development of contrast-induced nephropathy after percutaneous coronary interventions in patients with stable angina and normal serum creatinine values? *Kidney Blood Press Res* 2007;30:408–15.

In: Neutrophil Gelatinase-Associated Lipocalin   ISBN: 978-1-63117-984-6
Editors: M. Hur and S. Di Somma   © 2014 Nova Science Publishers, Inc.

Chapter 14

NGAL in Acute Heart Failure Patients

*Fatima Iqbal[*1], Hermineh Aramin[1], Minal V. Patel[1],*
Matt Kawahara[1], Sumita Sharma[1] and Alan S. Maisel[1,2]
[1]Veterans Affairs San Diego Healthcare System, San Diego, CA, US
[2]Department of Medicine, University of California at San Diego,
La Jolla,CA, US

Abstract

Acute kidney injury (AKI) represents a severe pathological condition common to many critical and potentially life-threatening diseases, such as acute heart failure (AHF), sepsis, hypovolemic shock, and contrast-induced nephropathy. Neutrophil gelatinase-associated lipocalin (NGAL) has been demonstrated to be a marker of AKI for many clinical conditions. Considering the multifactorial origin of HF and the fact that it is a fatal finishing line of all cardiovascular diseases (CVDs), there has been a quest for efficient diagnostic and prognostic biomarkers of HF to help design a scheme to optimize risk stratification of AHF patients and potentially improve preventive and therapeutic approaches. Obtaining NGAL levels in AHF patients, in addition to the well-documented markers BNP/NT-proBNP, will certainly help the clinicians to early manifest and intervene, as early treatment strategies, may have an impact

[*] correspondence: fatima@hotmail.com.

on clinical outcomes such as reduction in intensive care unit stay, hospital stay, morbidity, and mortality.

Introduction

Treatment and disposition decision making for patients with acute heart failure (AHF) represents one of the foremost difficulties for any physician. AHF patients often have variable co-morbidities that influence responses to therapy and post-treatment outcomes, complicating the decision of whether to discharge or admit. Deterioration of renal function is a prevalent complication of AHF exacerbation and is the most challenging of these co-morbidities [1 - 3]. In the past few decades, cardiovascular research has revolutionized the treatment, management, and prevention of arrhythmias, valvular diseases, congenital heart disease, and transplants via medication, prosthetics and biomedical instruments such as echocardiograms; however, the same cannot be said for heart failure (HF).

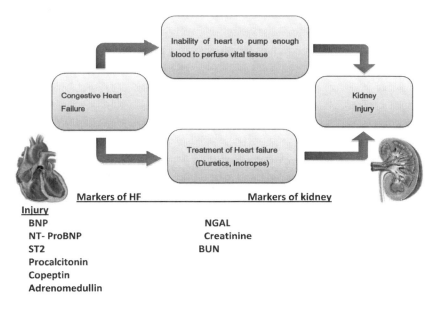

Figure 1. Schematic representation of the consequences of AHF and its treatment (esp. diuretics) on the kidneys. NGAL is a novel biomarker of kidney injury and has been shown to be elevated in patients with acute and chronic HF. In addition to other biomarkers of HF, such as BNP, NT-proBNP, adrenomedullin, ST2, copeptin, and procalcitonin, NGAL has shown an association between cardiac and renal damages.

The kidney and heart are substantially affected by pathology of each other. Cardio-renal syndrome (CRS) is an umbrella term for this condition, whereby "acute or chronic dysfunction in one organ may induce acute or chronic dysfunction of the other" (Fig. 1) [4].

In order to better consider kidney function, many markers have been suggested of which neutrophil gelatinase-associated lipocalin (NGAL) appears to have garnered much attention [4].

NGAL is predominantly expressed in tubular injury and is considered a better marker for predicting acute kidney injury (AKI) than plasma creatinine. Circulating NGAL in the serum is filtered by glomerulus, and then reabsorbed by proximal tubule [5]. Recent research has demonstrated the potential of NGAL as a diagnostic and prognostic marker of predicting worsening renal outcomes in patients with acute or chronic HF as well. It has been shown that both plasma and urinary NGAL levels are early predictors of AKI in a number of distinct clinical settings, such as post-cardiac surgery, kidney transplantation, contrast nephropathy, and HF [6 - 11]. These investigations proposed an association between elevated serum/urine NGAL levels and the development of both worsening renal failure and subsequent adverse events at 30 – 90 days after emergency department (ED) presentation [12]. As a result of recent research, NGAL has evolved as a diagnostic and prognostic tool for risk stratifying patients with HF and cardiovascular diseases (CVD).

Epidemiology and Clinical Development of NGAL

NGAL, also known as (human neutrophil lipocalin, lipocalin-2, siderocalin, 24p3, or LCN2) is a member of the lipocalin family of proteins. Human NGAL was first purified and recognized in 1993 by Kjeldsen et al. [13]. NGAL is a 25-kDa glycoprotein of 178 amino acids with a beta barrel structure and a hydrophobic ligand core. Most importantly, it has the ability to bind siderophores that function as iron-transport proteins as well as to prevent iron-mediated cell toxicity via endocytosis at the proximal tubule [13]. NGAL has been shown to be involved in immune modulation, inflammation and neoplastic transformation through macromolecule complexing and expression in immature neutrophils and epithelial cells [14, 15]. Broadly speaking, NGAL is rapidly released by a variety of cell types in the lung, kidney, trachea, stomach, and colon.

Studies done in the past on NGAL used animal models to clarify its potential role as a biomarker of AKI [16 - 18]. Numerous clinical trials done on NGAL have demonstrated its superiority over creatinine in predicting AKI and have also validated its use as a predictive marker of chronic kidney disease (CKD) [19 - 21]. Aghel et al. [22] measured plasma NGAL levels in hospitalized acute decompensated heart failure (ADHF) patients. Thirty-five patients (38%) developed WRF within the 5-day follow-up. Patients who developed WRF versus those without WRF had significantly higher median admission serum NGAL levels ($P = 0.001$). High serum NGAL levels on admission were associated with greater likelihood of developing WRF ($P = 0.004$). This study demonstrated that increased serum NGAL levels on admission are associated with profound risk of subsequent development of WRF in patients admitted with ADHF.

When the heart fails, there is activation of numerous immune and inflammatory mediators, particularly involving neutrophils, cardiomyocytes, and fibroblasts. This process is also associated with increased NGAL mRNA expression and protein concentrations. Patients with MI have cardiomyocyte damage resulting in ventricular remodeling and subsequent development of left ventricular dysfunction, precipitating acute and chronic HF. Yndestad et al. [23] demonstrated that in patients with acute post-MI HF and chronic HF, there was enhanced systemic and myocardial NGAL expression that correlated with clinical and neurohormonal deterioration. This study also demonstrated that components of the innate immune system were potential inducers of NGAL expression in failing cardiomyocytes.

The efficacy of NGAL in CVD revolves around its role in the ongoing inflammatory process that occurs in atherosclerotic plaques. NGAL is involved in protein breakdown, plaque disruption, and ventricular remodeling in patients presenting with progressive atherosclerotic disease, who are at risk for MI as well as progression to post-MI HF. Further studies are required in order to better understand the exact role of NGAL in failing myocardium using larger patient cohorts and testing composite endpoints.

Validation and Clinical Studies

NGAL, an established marker of renal injury, recently has gained the status of a novel cardiovascular risk predictor in patients with AHF. Data suggest that elevated NGAL levels after AHF management serves as an early marker for WRF and outcomes (Fig. 1). Moreover, there is compelling evidence of its increasingly distinct role in diagnosis and prognosis of HF patients. Alvelos et al. [26] studied the role of NGAL in prognostic stratification of HF patients. They reported that serum NGAL is an independent predictor of worse short-term prognosis in patients with AHF. Furthermore, it is impressive to know that serum NGAL levels of > 167.5 ng/mL was associated with almost threefold increase in risk of death and rehospitalization within 90 days of admission for AHF.

Evidence also suggests the potential utility of NGAL in staging patients with regards to their cardiovascular risk. Bolignano et al. [27] conducted a study on 46 patients with different severity of CHF and followed them for 2 years. Markedly increased levels of NGAL were found in these patients in comparison to age-matched healthy control population. Furthermore, these levels presented a clear correlation in accordance to NYHA class ($P = 0.0001$), with the levels of systolic pressure ($P = 0.05$), cholesterolemia ($P = 0.04$), albuminuria ($P = 0.05$) and ejection fraction ($P = 0.05$). They also observed that individuals whose baseline NGAL levels were > 783 ng/mL had a higher mortality rate, thus confirming NGAL as a useful tool for stratifying the patients according to their mortality risk during a 2-year follow-up period.

NGAL cannot only be detected in blood but it can be easily measured in urine making it a convenient protein that can be measured in different clinical settings [28]. AKI is a complication not infrequently seen after cardiac procedures and in critically ill patients. Torregrosa *et al.* [29] demonstrated that urine NGAL is an early marker for diagnosing AKI in patients presenting with acute coronary syndrome (ACS) or HF and undergoing cardiac surgery and coronary angiography ($P < 0.001$), having a predictive power superior to cystatin C and interleukin-18 (IL-18).

NGAL was studied in numerous other cardiovascular conditions such as atherosclerosis and ACS with good results that may impact screening, intervention, and prevention. Rancho Bernardo study [30] pointed that higher NGAL levels remained an independent predictor of all-cause mortality, (HR = 1.19, 95% confidence interval [CI]: 1.07 - 1.32), CVD mortality (HR = 1.33, 95% CI: 1.12 - 1.57), and a combined cardiovascular endpoint (HR = 1.26, 95% CI: 1.10 - 1.45) in community dwelling, older adults. Moreover, it adds complementary information to NT-proBNP and CRP (Fig. 2).

Kaplan-Meier curves based on NGAL and NT-proBNP levels above or below the median (192 ng/mL for NGAL, and 111 pg/mL for NT-proBNP). Four groups are compared: those with both NGAL and NT-proBNP below the median (n = 380; 57 deaths, 12 cardiovascular; 38 combined endpoint occurrences), those with only NGAL above the median (n = 316; 67 deaths, 20 cardiovascular; 40 combined endpoint occurrences), those with only NT-proBNP above the median (n = 316; 104 deaths, 43 cardiovascular; 56 combined endpoint occurrences), and those with both markers above the median (n = 378; 207 deaths, 93 cardiovascular; 119 combined endpoint occurrences). Three participants did not have NT-proBNP measured. Log rank $P < 0.001$ for each. A) CVD death. B) All-cause mortality. C) Combined cardiovascular endpoint (coronary revascularization, myocardial infarction, or CVD death). *Adapted from [30] with permission of Elsevier Inc.*

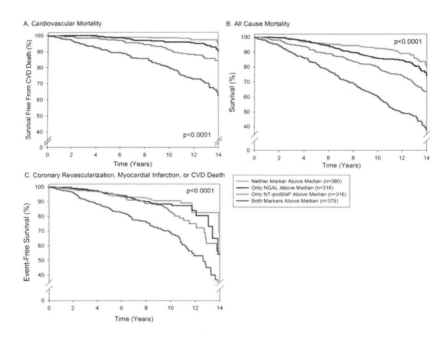

Figure 2. Combination of NGAL and NT-proBNP and Risk of Death or CVD.

Biomarker Guided/Multimarker Strategy

Reducing patient hospitalization and mortality due to AHF is of great importance. However, the ability to efficiently and accurately diagnose a patient with AHF has historically been a daunting task. HF is considered to be the final result of a culmination of cardiovascular disorders and comorbidities. Each biomarker plays a specific role in the attempt to identify these pathophysiological abnormalities that characterize HF. In conjunction with clinical evaluations, biomarkers offer an objective method of supplementing diagnostic and prognostic accuracy. Because of the specificity of AHF biomarkers, a single diagnostic test is not realistic for the identification of AHF. Therefore, a multi-marker approach is required to establish an accurate assessment of a patient with AHF [31, 32].

Table 1. Alternative biomarkers in heart failure

Biomarker	Description	Diagnostic/Prognostic Value
BNP	B-type natriuretic peptide, a 32 amino acid molecule, is released from myocytes under strain [31]. Levels will increase in response to abnormal cardiac dilation, increased fluid volume, and increased left ventricular preload [32].	A BNP level of 100 pg/mL has been found to have an 83% diagnostic accuracy for AHF [33]. Higher BNP levels on admission have been correlated with higher rates of in-hospital mortality. Lower readmission rates and lower in-hospital mortality have been observed with BNP guided therapy for AHF. Using BNP in conjunction with NGAL provides excellent risk stratification [33].
NT-proBNP	N-terminal prohormone of BNP, 76 amino acids in length, comes from the same precursor as BNP and is also released by strained cardiac myocytes [32].	NT-proBNP cutoff levels for AHF [34] are strongly based on patients' age. For patients < 50 years old, a cutoff of 450 pg/mL has been shown to have diagnostic accuracy of 95%. For patients >50 years old, a cutoff of 900 pg/mL has been shown to have diagnostic accuracy of 85%. The longer half-life of NT-proBNP may allow for better indication of ventricular stress in AHF [34].
ST2	ST2 is an inflammatory cytokine and belongs to the interleukin-1family of receptors. It is secreted in response to myocyte stretch. Elevated ST2 levels are seen in patients with severe AHF [32].	While the diagnostic value of ST2 is still under examination, ST2 has been shown to be a predictor of death and HF, especially in patients presenting with STEMI [35]. Supplementary to other biomarkers, ST2 can be useful in HF prognostication [32].
Procalcitonin	Procalcitonin is a 116 amino acid peptide produced by thyroidal c-cells. It is useful in the detection of bacterial infection; elevated levels can be observed when infection is present [31].	Procalcitonin can identify underlying bacterial infection more effectively than chest x-ray and blood testing [32]. Maisel et al. [36] showed that patients with AHF and pneumonia had median procalcitonin levels of 0.18 ng/mL; those without pneumonia showed median levels of 0.07 ng/mL. The correlation between procalcitonin concentration and infection severity suggests that procalcitonin-guided administration of antibiotics can help improve survival in these patients.

Table 1. (Continued)

Biomarker	Description	Diagnostic/Prognostic Value
CRP	C-reactive protein is an inflammatory biomarker produced in the liver. CRP is associated with cardiovascular risk [32].	CRP can be useful in helping to predict cardiovascular risk and HF. However, it lacks specificity which makes its diagnostic value very limited [32].
Copeptin	Copeptin is a surrogate marker of arginine vasopressin (AVP); it is generally more stable and robust than AVP [32]. Its concentration has been correlated with negative outcomes in patients with AHF [32].	Studies have shown that copeptin has high prognostic value in AHF patients. Higher levels were observed to predict negative outcomes including mortality and readmission [37].
MR-proANP	Mid-regional pro A-type natriuretic peptide is the epitope of the ANP prohormone [38]. MR-proANP has shown to be a robust and reliable analyte in the detection and risk stratification of AHF [39].	The BACH trial [39] has shown that MR-proANP can provide additional diagnostic information when other natriuretic peptide testing is unclear. The diagnostic power of MR-proANP is equivalent to BNP and NT-proBNP.
MR-proADM	Mid-regional pro-adrenomedullin is a peptide of the adrenomedullin (ADM) precursor and regulates volume and electrolyte homeostasis.	Results of the BACH trial [39] suggest that the prognostic power of MR-proADM is superior to that of BNP or NT-proBNP. Klip et al. [40] showed that those with developing HF and high levels of MR-proADM were up to three times more likely to predict all-cause mortality.

Natriuretic peptides have been instrumental in differentiating patients presenting in the ED with cardiac dyspnea versus non-cardiac dyspnea further aiding AHF diagnosis. NGAL, initially an AKI biomarker, has been shown to be useful in the prediction of negative AHF outcomes. Additionally, in the GALLANT study [41], NGAL and BNP were used together demonstrating prognostic power greater than what the biomarkers would obtain individually. Procalcitonin, copeptin, ST2, and NT-proBNP are additional markers that have shown evidence of diagnostic and prognostic value [31, 32]. Procalcitonin is useful in identifying underlying infections such as pneumonia in AHF patients [31, 32]. Copeptin is a newer marker, which has also shown potential in the assessment of patients with AHF. Using these novel markers in a multi-marker approach for diagnosis, prognosis and even biomarker-guided treatment shows promise in reducing the rates of negative outcomes in patients with AHF (Table 1).

Areas of Critique and Future Direction

A turning point in the new focus of NGAL, a promising nephrology biomarker, is its interesting involvement in the clinical field of CVDs, such as the pathogenesis and clinical manifestations of atherosclerosis, acute myocardial infarction (MI) and heart failure.

Evidence suggests the role of NGAL in the progression of CAD to MI. Elevated NGAL levels is found in atherosclerotic plaques, where it is responsible for augmenting the inflammatory process leading to plaque disruption resulting in MI. Although it appears reasonable to assume that NGAL is markedly hyperexpressed by the damaged myocardium and it may be considered an active mediator in post-ischemic inflammation and remodeling responses [23, 42], yet, confounding factors such as hypertension, inflammation, anemia, and existing cancer may also influence plasma NGAL levels. However, as with any novel biomarker, limitations in NGAL properties do exist.

Recent studies have revealed that NGAL is involved in CVDs and its complications. Now the question arises whether NGAL represents an important link between renal and cardiovascular function and it can be included in the panel of biomarkers of the cardio-renal axis. The best way to obtain a pragmatic answer to the current information overload about NGAL and clearly define its efficacy and instructions for use in daily clinical practice requires further quality-improved multicenter studies.

Conclusion

Considering the multifactorial origin of HF and the fact that it is a fatal finishing line of all CVDs, there has been a quest for efficient diagnostic and prognostic biomarkers of HF to help design a scheme to optimize risk stratification of AHF patients and potentially improve preventive and therapeutic approaches. Reliable detectors of deteriorating renal function in

ED patients with AHF are limited. The presumption of a causal linkage between AHF and WRF and subsequent outcomes, or the categorization of renal impairment as an important clinical outcome in its own right, has led to the exploration of markers that depict kidney injury in the setting of ADHF. Obtaining NGAL levels in the ED especially in AHF patients, in addition to the well-documented markers BNP/NT-ProBNP, will certainly help the clinicians to early manifest and intervene, as early treatment strategies, may have an impact on clinical outcomes such as reduction in intensive care unit stay, hospital stay, morbidity, and mortality.

References

[1]   Gottlieb SS, Abraham W, Butler J, Forman DE, Loh E, Massie BM, O'connor CM, Rich MW, Stevenson LW, Young J, Krumholz HM. The prognostic importance of different definitions of worsening renal function in congestive heart failure. *J Card Fail* 2002;8:136-41.

[2]   Fonarow GC, Adams KF Jr, Abraham WT, Yancy CW, Boscardin WJ. Risk stratification for in-hospital mortality in acutely decompensated heart failure: classification and regression tree analysis. *JAMA* 2005;293:572-80.

[3]   Collins SP, Lindsell CJ, Naftilan AJ, Peacock WF, Diercks D, Hiestand B, Maisel A, Storrow AB. Low-risk acute heart failure patients: external validation of the Society of Chest Pain Center's recommendations. *Crit Pathw Cardiol* 2009;8:99-103.

[4]   Ronco C, Haapio M, House AA, Anavekar N, Bellomo R. Cardio-renal syndrome. *J Am Coll Cardiol* 2008;52:1527-39.

[5]   Schmidt-Ott KM, Mori K, Li JY, Kalandadze A, Cohen DJ, Devarajan P, Barasch J. Dual action of neutrophil gelatinase-associated lipocalin. *J Am Soc Nephrol* 2007;18:407-13.

[6]   Haase M, Devarajan P, Haase-Fielitz A, Bellomo R, Cruz DN, Wagener G, Krawczeski CD, Koyner JL, Murray P, Zappitelli M, Goldstein SL, Makris K, Ronco C, Martensson J, Martling CR, Venge P, Siew E, Ware LB, Ikizler TA, Mertens PR. The outcome of neutrophil gelatinase-associated lipocalin-positive subclinical acute kidney injury: a multicenter pooled analysis of prospective studies. *J Am Coll Cardiol* 2011;57: 1752-61.

[7]   Mishra J, Dent C, Tarabishi R, Mitsnefes MM, Ma Q, Kelly C, Ruff SM, Zahedi K, Shao M, Bean J, Mori K, Barasch J, Devarajan P. Neutrophil

gelatinase-associated lipocalin (NGAL) as a biomarker for acute renal injury after cardiac surgery. *Lancet* 2005;365:1231-8.

[8] Nickolas TL, O'Rourke MJ, Yang J, Sise ME, Canetta PA, Barasch N, Buchen C, Khan F, Mori K, Giglio J, Devarajan P, Barasch J. Sensitivity and specificity of a single emergency department measurement of urinary neutrophil gelatinase-associated lipocalin for diagnosing acute kidney injury. *Ann Intern Med* 2008;148: 810-9.

[9] Siew ED, Ware LB, Gebretsadik T, Shintani A, Moons KG, Wickersham N, Bossert F, Ikizler TA. Urine neutrophil gelatinase-associated lipocalin moderately predicts acute kidney injury in critically ill adults. *J Am Soc Nephrol* 2009;20:1823-32.

[10] Hollmen ME, Kyllonen LE, Inkinen KA, Lalla ML, Salmela KT. Urine neutrophil gelatinase-associated lipocalin is a marker of graft recovery after kidney transplantation. *Kidney Int* 2011;79:89-98.

[11] Bachorzewska-Gajewska H, Malyszko J, Sitniewska E, Malyszko JS, Dobrzycki S. Neutrophil gelatinase-associated lipocalin (NGAL) correlations with cystatin C, serum creatinine. *Nephrol Dial Transplant* 2007; 22:295-6.

[12] Shemin D, Dworkin LD. Neutrophil gelatinase-associated lipocalin (NGAL) as a biomarker for early acute kidney injury. Crit Care Clin 2011;27:379-89.

[13] Kjeldsen L, Johnsen AH, Sengeløv H, Borregaard N. Isolation and primary structure of NGAL, a novel protein associated with human neutrophil gelatinase. *J Biol Chem* 1993;268:10425-32.

[14] Flower DR. The lipocalin protein family: structure and function. *Biochem J* 1996;318:1-14.

[15] Goetz DH, Willie ST, Armen RS, Bratt T, Borregaard N, Strong RK. Ligand preference inferred from the structure of neutrophil gelatinase associated lipocalin. *Biochemistry* 2000;39:1935-41.

[16] Mori K, Lee HT, Rapoport D, Drexler IR, Foster K, Yang J, Schmidt-Ott KM, Chen X, Li JY, Weiss S, Mishra J, Cheema FH, Markowitz G, Suganami T, Sawai K, Mukoyama M, Kunis C, D'Agati V, Devarajan P, Barasch J. Endocytic delivery of lipocalin-siderophore-iron complex rescues the kidney from ischemia-reperfusion injury. *J Clin Invest* 2005;115: 610-21.

[17] Mishra J, Mori K, Ma Q. Amelioration of ischemic acute renal injury by neutrophil gelatinase-associated lipocalin. *J Am Soc Nephrol* 2004;15:3073-82.

[18] Mishra J, Ma Q, Prada A, Mitsnefes M, Zahedi K, Yang J, Barasch J, Devarajan P. Identification of NGAL as a novel early urinary marker for ischemic renal injury. *J Am Soc Nephrol* 2003;14:2534-43.

[19] Zappitelli M, Washburn KK, Arikan AA, Loftis L, Ma Q, Devarajan P, Parikh CR, Goldstein SL. Urine neutrophil gelatinase-associated lipocalin is an early marker of acute kidney injury in critically ill children: a prospective cohort study. *Crit Care* 2007;11:R84.

[20] Makris K, Markou N, Evodia E. Urinary neutrophil gelatinase-associated lipocalin (NGAL) as an early marker of acute kidney injury in critically ill multiple trauma patients. *Clin Chem Lab Med* 2009;47:79-82.

[21] de Geus HR, Bakker J, Lesaffre EM, le Noble JL. Neutrophil gelatinase-associated lipocalin at ICU admission predicts for acute kidney injury in adult patients. *Am J Respir Crit Care Med* 2011;183:907-14.

[22] Aghel A, Shrestha K, Mullens W, Borowski A, Tang WH. Serum neutrophil gelatinase-associated lipocalin (NGAL) in predicting worsening renal function in acute decompensated heart failure. *J Card Fail* 2010;16:49-54.

[23] Yndestad A, Landrø L, Ueland T, Dahl CP, Flo TH, Vinge LE, Espevik T, Frøland SS, Husberg C, Christensen G, Dickstein K, Kjekshus J, Øie E, Gullestad L, Aukrust P. Increased systemic and myocardial expression of neutrophil gelatinase-associated lipocalin in clinical and experimental heart failure. *Eur J Heart Fail* 2009;30:1229-36.

[24] Bolignano D, Lacquaniti A, Coppolino G, Donato V, Campo S, Fazio MR, Nicocia G, Buemi M. Neutrophil Gelatinase-Associated Lipocalin (NGAL) and progression of chronic kidney disease. *Clin J Am Soc Nephrol* 2009;4:337-44.

[25] Mitsnefes M, Kathman T, Mishra J. Serum neutrophil gelatinase-associated lipocalin as a marker of renal function in children with chronic kidney disease. *Pediatric Nephrol* 2007;22: 101-8.

[26] Alvelos M, Lourenco P, Dias C, Amorim M, Rema J, Leite AB, Guimarães JT, Almeida P, Bettencourt P. Prognostic value of neutrophil gelatinase associated lipocalin in acute heart failure. *Int J Cardiol* 2013; 165:51-5.

[27] Bolignano D, Basile G, Parisi P, Coppolino G, Nicocia G, Buemi M. Increased plasma neutrophil gelatinase-associated lipocalin levels predict mortality in elderly patients with chronic heart failure. *Rejuvenation Res* 2009;12:7–14.

[28] Hawkins R. New biomarkers of acute kidney injury and the cardio-renal syndrome. *Korean J Lab Med* 2011;31:72-80.

[29] Torregrosa I, Montoliu C, Urios A, Elmlili N, Puchades MJ, Solís MA, Sanjuán R, Blasco ML, Ramos C, Tomás P, Ribes J, Carratalá A, Juan I, Miguel A. Early biomarkers of acute kidney failure after heart angiography or heart surgery in patients with acute coronary syndrome or acute heart failure. *Nefrologia* 2012;32:44-52.

[30] Daniels LB, Barrett-Connor E, Clopton P, Laughlin GA, Ix JH, Maisel AS. Plasma neutrophil gelatinase-associated lipocalin is independently associated with cardiovascular disease and mortality in community-dwelling older adults: the Rancho Bernardo study. *J Am Coll Cardiol* 2012;59:1101-9.

[31] Choudhary R, Di Somma S, Maisel AS. Biomarkers for diagnosis and prognosis of acute heart failure. *Curr Em Hosp Med Rep* 2013;1:133-40.

[32] Iqbal N, Wentworth B., Choudhary R., Landa Ade L, Kipper B, Fard A, Maisel AS. Cardiac biomarkers: new tools for heart failure management. *Cardiovasc Diagn Ther* 2012;2:147-64.

[33] Maisel AS, Krishnaswamy P, Nowak RM, McCord J, Hollander JE, Duc P, Omland T, Storrow AB, Abraham WT, Wu AH, Clopton P, Steg PG, Westheim A, Knudsen CW, Perez A, Kazanegra R, Herrmann HC, McCullough PA; Breathing Not Properly Multinational Study Investigators. Rapid measurement of B-type natriuretic peptide in the emergency diagnosis of heart failure. *N Engl J Med* 2002;347:161-7.

[34] Januzzi JL Jr, Camargo CA, Anwaruddin S, Baggish AL, Chen AA, Krauser DG, Tung R, Cameron R, Nagurney JT, Chae CU, Lloyd-Jones DM, Brown DF, Foran-Melanson S, Sluss PM, Lee-Lewandrowski E, Lewandrowski KB. The N-terminal pro-BNP investigation of dyspnea in the emergency department (PRIDE) study. *Am J Cardiol* 2005;95:948-54.

[35] Shimpo M, Morrow DA, Weinberg EO, Sabatine MS, Murphy SA, Antman EM, Lee RT. Serum levels of the Interleukin-1 receptor family member ST2 predict mortality and clinical outcome in acute myocardial infarction. *Circulation* 2004;109:2186-90.

[36] Maisel A, Neath SX, Landsberg J, Mueller C, Nowak RM, Peacock WF, Ponikowski P, Möckel M, Hogan C, Wu AH, Richards M, Clopton P, Filippatos GS, Di Somma S, Anand I, Ng LL, Daniels LB, Christenson RH, Potocki M, McCord J, Terracciano G, Hartmann O, Bergmann A, Morgenthaler NG, Anker SD. Use of procalcitonin for the diagnosis of

pneumonia in patients presenting with a chief complaint of dyspnea: results from the BACH (biomarkers in acute heart failure) trial. *Eur J Heart Fail* 2012;14:278-86.

[37] Maisel A, Xue Y, Shah K, Mueller C, Nowak R, Peacock WF, Ponikowski P, Mockel M, Hogan C, Wu AH, Richards M, Clopton P, Filippatos GS, Di Somma S, Anand IS, Ng L, Daniels LB, Neath SX, Christenson R, Potocki M, McCord J, Terracciano G, Kremastinos D, Hartmann O, von Haehling S, Bergmann A, Morgenthaler NG, Anker SD. Increased 90-day mortality in patients with acute heart failure with elevated copeptin: secondary results from the Biomarkers in Acute Heart Failure (BACH) study. *Circ Heart Fail* 2011;4:613-20.

[38] Morgenthaler NG Struck J, Thomas B, Bergmann A. Immunoluminometric assay for the midregion of pro-atrial natriuretic peptide in human plasma. *Clin Chem* 2004;50:234-6.

[39] Maisel A, Mueller C, Nowak R, Peacock WF, Landsberg JW, Ponikowski P, Mockel M, Hogan C, Wu AH, Richards M, Clopton P, Filippatos GS, Di Somma S, Anand I, Ng L, Daniels LB, Neath SX, Christenson R, Potocki M, McCord J, Terracciano G, Kremastinos D, Hartmann O, von Haehling S, Bergmann A, Morgenthaler NG, Anker SD. Mid-region pro-hormone markers for diagnosis and prognosis in acute dyspnea: Results from the BACH (Biomarkers in Acute Heart Failure) trial. *J Am Coll Cardiol* 2010;55:2062-76.

[40] Klip IT, Voors AA, Anker SD, Hillege HL, Struck J, Squire I, van Veldhuisen DJ, Dickstein K; OPTIMAAL investigators. Prognostic value of mid-regional pro-adrenomedullin in patients with HF after an acute myocardial infarction. *Heart* 2011;97:892-8.

[41] Maisel AS, Mueller C, Fitzgerald R, Brikhan R, Hiestand BC, Iqbal N, Clopton P, van Veldhuisen DJ. Prognostic utility of plasma neutrophil gelatinase-associated lipocalin in patients with acute heart failure: the NGAL evaluation along with b-type natriuretic peptide in acutely decompensated heart failure (GALLANT) trial. *Eur J Heart Fail* 2011;13:846-51.

[42] Hemdahl AL, Gabrielsen A, Zhu C, Eriksson P, Hedin U, Kastrup J,Thorén P, Hansson GK. Expression of neutrophil gelatinase-associated lipocalin in atherosclerosis and myocardial infarction. *Arterioscler Thromb Vasc Biol* 2006;26:136–42.

In: Neutrophil Gelatinase-Associated Lipocalin   ISBN: 978-1-63117-984-6
Editors: M. Hur and S. Di Somma   © 2014 Nova Science Publishers, Inc.

Chapter 15

NGAL in Septic Patients

Laura Magrini[*1], Benedetta De Berardinis[1], Mina Hur[2] and Salvatore Di Somma[1]*

[1]Department of Medical-Surgery Sciences and Translational Medicine,
University Sapienza Rome, Emergency Department Emergency Medicine
Sant'Andrea Hospital, Rome, Italy
[2]Department of Laboratory Medicine,
Konkuk University School of Medicine, Seoul, Korea

Abstract

Acute kidney injury (AKI) represents a severe pathological condition common to many critical and potentially life-threatening diseases, such as acute heart failure, sepsis, hypovolemic shock, and contrast-induced nephropathy. Serum creatinine takes more than 48 hours to detect the occurrence of AKI and should not be considered an early marker of AKI for these patients. As a consequence, it seems necessary to have a specific and sensitive biomarker, faster than serum creatinine, for the early detection of AKI in order to stop the progression of renal failure in these critical illnesses. The use of NGAL seems to be very useful in the management of septic patients; it permits early diagnosis of early AKI and prognostic risk stratification for death. This could lead in the future to an NGAL driven antibiotic therapy to prevent AKI in patients with sepsis and AKI.

[*] correspondence: magrinilau@libero.it.

Introduction

Sepsis, a systemic inflammatory response syndrome associated with signs and symptoms of infectious disease [1], is one of the first causes of morbidity and mortality in critically ill patients [2]. For these patients, mortality rates range from 20% for sepsis, to 40% for severe sepsis and to 60% for septic shock [3]. Sepsis is the major contributing factor for the development of AKI. The relation between sepsis and AKI is not completely understood, it is considered to be associated with pathophysiological alterations linked to septic disease, such as microvessel thrombosis, hypoperfusion, infiltration of immune cells, and apoptosis [4, 5].

A number of novel biomarkers have been recently developed for earlier and more specific detection of AKI; neutrophil gelatinase-associated lipocalin (NGAL) is one of them. Elevated serum NGAL levels were previously found to identify bacterial infections in non-critically ill children and adults [6, 7]. Only during the last decade, focus shifted and NGAL has become a promising marker for early detection of AKI.

NGAL is expressed in epithelial cells under inflammatory conditions [8]; nevertheless a variety of other functions has been reported for NGAL, such as induction of apoptosis in cytokine-dependent neutrophils and other leukocytes [9], suppression of bacterial growth [10], and modulation of inflammatory responses. NGAL might also be a scavenger of bacterial products at sites of inflammation [11].

In consideration of pathogenesis of septic AKI, a long-held paradigm considered that septic AKI is primary due to reduced renal blood flow, renal vasoconstriction in response to decrease perfusion, tubular cell hypoxia, bioenergetic failure and cell death. [12-14]. Actually, a growing body of experimental data support notion that immune-mediated injury and apoptosis are strongly involved in the pathogenesis of septic AKI in an independent way from decrease of renal perfusion [13]. Moreover, observational data suggest that in septic patients a delay in an appropriate antibiotic therapy is a relevant independent factor associated with a higher risk for AKI [15].

NGAL in Septic AKI

In septic AKI, the diagnostic value of NGAL is strongly influenced by different reasons: 1) NGAL is produced not only by tubular cells of kidney; 2) directly secreted by activated neutrophils. For this reason, plasma NGAL might reflect sepsis severity rather than AKI per se. Martensson et al. [16] recently demonstrated that rise of plasma NGAL in non AKI patients with systemic inflammatory response syndrome (SIRS) further increases with sepsis severity. Two different immunoassays that can distinguish the monomeric form of NGAL (mainly released by kidney epithelial cells) from the dimeric form (mainly released by activated neutrophils) have been recently tested. These two assays could be really useful in the future in distinguishing the origin of NGAL release [17].

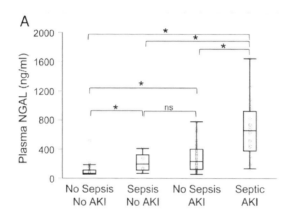

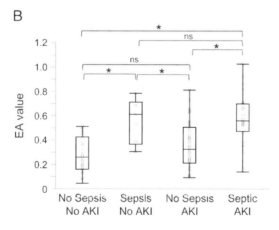

Figure 1. Plasma NGAL and endotoxin activity (EA) levels. Plasma NGAL measurement and EA were performed in adult ICU patients. Nonseptic non-AKI (n = 40), septic non-AKI (n = 10), nonseptic AKI (n = 65), and septic AKI (n = 24). *P < 0.05. Adapted from [19] with permission of Elsevier Inc.

The first study of the role of plasma NGAL in septic patients was published by Shapiro et al. [18]. They demonstrated that, in patients with suspected sepsis, increased NGAL concentration measured at the time of presentation to the ED were associated with the development of AKI. Recently Katagiri et al. [19] showed that in intensive care unit (ICU), septic AKI can be detected reliably by measurement of plasma NGAL that was significantly higher in septic AKI patients than in the other AKI patients, and in non AKI patients (Fig. 1). The same findings were also shown in the study by Camou et al. [20]. They also showed the importance of serial assessment of plasma NGAL in septic AKI.

Bagshaw et al. [21] showed that septic AKI is very common during the first 24h after hospitalization, and this condition seems to be independently associated with higher risk of longer in-hospital stay. Shapiro et al. [22] formulated a septic score by creating a panel of three biomarkers (included NGAL) that was predictive not only of severe sepsis, septic shock, but also of death.

Conclusion

The use of NGAL seems to be very useful in the management of septic patients; it permits early diagnosis of early AKI and prognostic risk stratification for death. This could lead in the future to an NGAL driven antibiotic therapy to prevent AKI in patients with sepsis and AKI.

References

[1] Levy MM, Fink MP, Marshall JC, Abraham E, Angus D, Cook D, Cohen J, Opal SM, Vincent JL, Ramsay G; 2001 SCCM/ESICM/ACCP/ATS/SIS International Sepsis Definitions Conference. *Crit Care Med* 2003;31:1250-6.

[2] Lentini P, de Cal M, Clementi A, D'Angelo A, Ronco C. Sepsis and AKI in ICU Patients: The Role of Plasma Biomarkers. *Crit Care Res Pract* 2012;2012:856401.

[3] Brun-Buisson C. The epidemiology of the systemic inflammatory response. *Intens Care Med* 2000;26 Suppl 1:S64-74.

[4]   Payen D, Lukaszewicz AC, Legrand M, Gayat E, Faivre V, Megarbane B, Azoulay E, Fieux F, Charron D, Loiseau P, Busson M. A multicentre study of acute kidney injury in severe sepsis and septic shock: association with inflammatory phenotype and HLA genotype. *PLoS One PLoS One* 2012;7:e35838.

[5]   Lerolle N, Nochy D, Guérot E, Bruneval P, Fagon JY, Diehl JL, Hill G. Histopathology of septic shock induced acute kidney injury: apoptosis and leukocytic infiltration. *Intensive Care Med* 2010;36:471-8.

[6]   Fjaertoft G, Foucard T, Xu S, Venge P. Human neutrophil lipocalin (HNL) as a diagnostic tool in children with acute infections: a study of the kinetics. *Acta Paediatr* 2005;94:661-6.

[7]   Xu SY, Pauksen K, Venge P. Serum measurements of human neutrophil lipocalin (HNL) discriminate between acute bacterial and viral infections. *Scand J Clin Lab Invest* 1995;55:125-31.

[8]   Nielsen BS, Borregaard N, Bundgaard JR, Timshel S, Sehested M, Kjeldsen L. Induction of NGAL synthesis in epithelial cells of human colorectal neoplasia and inflammatory bowel diseases. *Gut* 1996;38:414-20.

[9]   Devireddy LR, Teodoro JG, Richard FA, Green MR. Induction of apoptosis by a secreted lipocalin that is transcriptionally regulated by IL-3 deprivation. *Science* 2001;293:829-34.

[10]   Goetz DH, Holmes MA, Borregaard N, Bluhm ME, Raymond KN, Strong RK. The neutrophil lipocalin NGAL is a bacteriostatic agent that interferes with siderophore-mediated iron acquisition. *Mol Cell* 2002;10:1033-43.

[11]   Nielsen BS,Borregaard N, Bundgaard JR, Timshel S, Sehested M, Kjeldsen L. Induction of NGAL synthesis in epithelial cells of human colorectal neoplasia and inflammatory bowel diseases. *Gut* 1996;38:414-20.

[12]   Bonventre JV. Pathophysiology of AKI: injury and normal and abnormal repair. *Contrib Nephrol* 2010;165:9-17.

[13]   Bellomo R, Wan L, Langenberg C, May C. Septic acute kidney injury: new concepts. *Nephron Exp Nephrol* 2008;109:c95-100.

[14]   Schrier RW, Wang W. Acute renal failure and sepsis. *N Engl J Med* 2004;351:159-69.

[15]   Bagshaw SM, Lapinsky S, Dial S, Arabi Y, Dodek P, Wood G, Ellis P, Guzman J, Marshall J, Parrillo JE, Skrobik Y, Kumar A; Cooperative Antimicrobial Therapy of Septic Shock (CATSS) Database Research Group. Acute kidney injury in septic shock: clinical outcomes and

impact of duration of hypotension prior to initiation of antimicrobial therapy. *Intensive Care Med* 2009;35:871-81.

[16] Mårtensson J, Bell M, Oldner A, Xu S, Venge P, Martling CR. Neutrophil gelatinase-associated lipocalin in adult septic patients with and without acute kidney injury. *Intensive Care Med* 2010;36:1333-4.

[17] Mårtensson J, Xu S, Bell M, Martling CR, Venge P. Immunoassays distinguishing between HNL/NGAL released in urine from kidney epithelial cells and neutrophils. *Clin Chim Acta* 2012;413:1661-7.

[18] Shapiro NI, Trzeciak S, Hollander JE, Birkhahn R, Otero R, Osborn TM, Moretti E, Nguyen HB, Gunnerson K, Milzman D, Gaieski DF, Goyal M, Cairns CB, Kupfer K, Lee SW, Rivers EP. The diagnostic accuracy of plasma neutrophil gelatinase-associated lipocalin in the prediction of acute kidney injury in emergency department patients with suspected sepsis. *Ann Emerg Med* 2010;56:52-9.

[19] Katagiri D, Doi K, Matsubara T, Negishi K, Hamasaki Y, Nakamura K, Ishii T, Yahagi N, Noiri E. New biomarker panel of plasma neutrophil gelatinase-associated lipocalin and endotoxin activity assay for detecting sepsis in acute kidney injury. *J Crit Care* 2013;28:564-70.

[20] Camou F, Oger S, Paroissin C, Guilhon E, Guisset O, Mourissoux G, Pouyes H, Lalanne T, Gabinski C. Plasma Neutrophil Gelatinase-Associated Lipocalin (NGAL) predicts acute kidney injury in septic shock at ICU admission. *Ann Fr Anesth Reanim* 2013;32:157-64.

[21] Bagshaw SM, George C, Bellomo R; ANZICS Database Management Committee. Early acute kidney injury and sepsis: a multicentre evaluation. *Crit Care* 2008;12:R47.

[22] Shapiro NI, Trzeciak S, Hollander JE, Birkhahn R, Otero R, Osborn TM, Moretti E, Nguyen HB, Gunnerson KJ, Milzman D, Gaieski DF, Goyal M, Cairns CB, Ngo L, Rivers EP. A prospective, multicenter derivation of a biomarker panel to assess risk of organ dysfunction, shock, and death in emergency department patients with suspected sepsis. *Crit Care Med* 2009;37:96-104.

In: Neutrophil Gelatinase-Associated Lipocalin   ISBN: 978-1-63117-984-6
Editors: M. Hur and S. Di Somma   © 2014 Nova Science Publishers, Inc.

Chapter 16

NGAL in Contrast-Induced Nephropathy

Benedetta De Berardinis[*], *Laura Magrini* *and Salvatore Di Somma*

Department of Medical-Surgery Sciences and Translational Medicine,
University Sapienza Rome, Emergency Department Emergency Medicine
Sant'Andrea Hospital, Rome, Italy

Abstract

Neutrophil gelatinase-associated lipocalin (NGAL) has been demonstrated to be a marker of acute kidney injury (AKI) for many clinical conditions. NGAL seems to be a robust and affordable biomarker for detection of AKI in patients with contrast-induced nephropathy (CIN). The studies published until now demonstrate the diagnostic value of NGAL to predict, earlier than cystatin C and serum creatinine, the onset of AKI in CIN. Prompt diagnosis of CIN is important to prevent AKI in CIN. The prolongation of length of stay, persistent kidney damage, renal failure requiring dialysis, and all-cause mortality in this pathological condition could be avoided by the use of NGAL. Serial measurements of NGAL in these patients should be recommended in order to optimize the efficacy of NGAL.

[*] Correspondence: benedetta.db@gmail.com.

Introduction

Contrast-induced nephropathy (CIN) is a clinical disease characterized by a decrease in glomerular filtration rate (GFR) as a consequence of iodinated contrast media (CM) injection. It is considered the third most common cause of in-hospital acute renal failure (ARF) (12%) after decreased renal perfusion (42%) and post-operative ARF (18%) [1].

Several routine radiographical diagnostic examinations, especially in acute settings, are CM-based and may therefore be complicated by CIN. The vast majority of CIN cases may be increasingly encountered after percutaneous coronary interventions (PCI) due to growing numbers of procedures. Moreover, the presence of multiple co-morbidities in patients undergoing PCI and larger amounts of CM used for complex coronary lesions could facilitate the occurrence of CIN.

Furthermore, CIN can develop after any radiographical contrast examinations, such as routine angiographic study included in computerized tomography (CT) scan.

Functionally, CIN is considered an intrinsic acute kidney injury (AKI), usually with preserved diuresis. Nevertheless, in severe cases, acute tubular necrosis and even end-stage renal disease may develop. As CIN is associated with disabling morbidity and mortality [2], prevention and early detection of CIN are of most clinical relevance [3, 4]. After intravascular CM injection, immediate renal toxicity may occur, and in most cases, it remains luckily free of significant clinical consequences. However, renal function can diminish and serum creatinine (sCr) may increase in the following days (Figure 1). In absence of a universally accepted definition [5], most authors define CIN as a relative ($\geq$ 25%) or an absolute ($\geq$ 0.5 mg/dL = 44 μmol/L) increase in sCr from baseline.

In the case of contrast-induced toxicity, sCr typically rises within the first 24 – 48 hours after exposure, peaks at 3 – 5 days and returns near to baseline within 1 – 3 weeks [6].

However, irreversible renal function losses may occur in rare cases. Obviously, in addition to CM exposure, the diagnosis of CIN requires (A) a temporal relationship between CM exposure and sCr elevation, and (B) the exclusion of an alternative cause to the ARF.

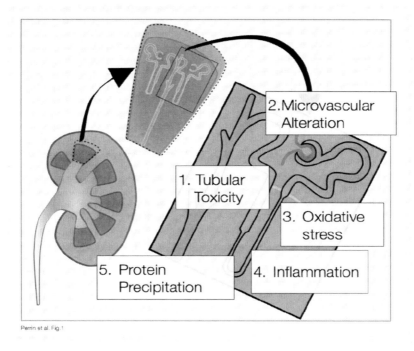

Figure 1. Schematic pathways contributing to the pathogenesis of CIN. *Adapted from [40] with permission from EMH Swiss Medical Publishers Ltd..*

Epidemiology and Prognosis

Considering the largest randomized controlled trials, evaluating the incidence of CIN following PCI during the last 5 years, protocol-defined CIN incidence ranged between < 1% to > 20%, with an increased incidence after emergency PCI [7 – 26]. A retrospective study on 5,967 all-comer patients with normal renal function undergoing PCI reported that both the 1-year myocardial infarction rate (24.0% vs. 11.6%, $P < 0.005$) and the 1-year mortality rate (9.5% vs. 2.7%, $P < 0.005$) were significantly higher in 208 patients (3.5%) who developed significant CIN. Similarly, in 439 patients with chronic renal failure undergoing PCI, Gruberg et al. [27] showed that 7% required transitory hemodialysis and 0.9% were discharged on chronic dialysis. Among the 161 (37%) patients developing CIN, there was a 2- to 3-fold increase in in-hospital (15% vs. 5%, $P = 0.001$) and 1-year mortality (35 – 45% vs. 19%, $P = 0.001$) in comparison to the patients without CIN. Finally, in an attempt to stratify the prognosis of patients who already developed CIN after PCI, Harjai et al. [28] proposed a 3-level scoring system (grade 0 [sCr < 25% and < 44 µmol/L], grade 1 [sCr ≥ 25% and < 44 µmol/L] and grade 2 [sCr ≥ 44 µmol/L]). They suggested that an increasing grade is correlated with a worse long-term outcome after PCI (6-month major adverse cardiac events [12.4 vs. 19.4 vs. 28.6%, $P = 0.003$]; 6-month all-cause mortality [10.2 vs. 10.4 vs. 40.9%, $P < 0.0001$]; n = 985).

Early Diagnosis

In order to minimize or stratify the risk of CIN, several scores have been proposed (Table 1) [29, 30]. Diagnosis of AKI in CIN relies on the monitoring of functional markers and/or biomarkers in serum and urine. To improve patient management, an ideal marker should be accurate and proportional to renal injury and have an early kinetic for mirroring acute renal damage. Moreover, it should help differentiate acute structural damage (AKI) from functional impairment (prerenal azotaemia) or chronic kidney disease (CKD). This is even more important as intrinsic ARF is linked with an increased risk of in-hospital mortality and/or need for dialysis [31]. In daily practice, changes in sCr are used to estimate acute modifications in renal function, and sCr monitoring remains the cornerstone for the diagnosis of CIN. Unfortunately, Cr is a late and insensitive indicator of acute changes in renal function, as there is a 4 − 48 hours delay between renal insult and sCr changes [32]. Because of this pitfall and since an early diagnosis may decrease morbidity and improve patient survival, accurate biomarkers are eagerly awaited for the early detection of tubular dysfunction/lesion [33]. Recently, NGAL has been demonstrated to be a promising biomarker of tubular insult due to CIN.

NGAL (Neutrophil Gelatinase - Associated Lipocalin)

In patients with chronic kidney disease, Alharazy et al. [34] demonstrated a predictive value of NGAL in diagnosing CIN after coronary angiography. They showed the usefulness of NGAL, greater than sCr, for the early diagnosis of CIN in patients who underwent coronary catheterization. Other studies have found a significant rise in serial assessment of both serum and urinary NGAL levels after PCI procedures [35 - 37]. They concluded that NGAL could represent a more sensitive and early biomarker of renal impairment in PCI more than other biomarkers as cystatin C. Ling et al. [38] also showed that urinary NGAL together with IL-18 were good early predictive biomarkers for detecting CIN after PCI. In patients with reduced renal filtration function undergoing coronary angiography, McCullough et al. [39] showed that NGAL level at baseline was strongly correlated with GFR. They also demonstrated that the magnitude of rise in NGAL was associated with the baseline level and its time course corresponded with that of sCr over the first 48 hours after contrast injection.

Table 1. Independent risk factors for contrast- induced nephropathy and calculation of Mehran simple risk score

CIN risk factors	Mehran simple risk – score definition [40]	Integer score
Decreased renal perfusion	Systolic blood pressure < 80 mm Hg for at least 1 h requiring support with medication or intra-aortic balloon pump within 24 h of the procedure	5
	Intra – aortic balloon pump within 24 h of the procedure	5
	Congestive heart failure class III or IV by the NYHA class and/or pulmonary edema	5
Older age	Age >75 years	4
Anemia	Baseline Hct < 39% for men and < 36% for women	3
Diabetes	Present or not	3
Contrast media volume	Absolute amount	1 for each 100 mL
Impaired baseline renal function	Baseline sCr > 1.5mg/dL or baseline eGFR < 60 mL/min	4 2 for 40 – 60 4 for 20 – 40 6 for < 20

Abbreviations: CIN, contrast- induced nephropathy; Hct, hematocrit; sCr, serum creatinine; eGFR, estimated glomerular filtration rate.

Conclusion

NGAL seems to be a robust and affordable biomarker for detection of AKI in patients with CIN. The studies published until now demonstrate the diagnostic value of NGAL to predict, earlier than cystatin C and sCr, the onset of AKI in CIN. Prompt diagnosis of CIN is important to prevent AKI in CIN. The prolongation of length of stay, persistent kidney damage, renal failure requiring dialysis, and all-cause mortality in this pathological condition could be avoided by the use of NGAL. Serial measurements of NGAL in these patients should be recommended in order to optimize the efficacy of NGAL.

References

[1]   Nash K, Hafeez A, Hou S. Hospital-acquired renal insufficiency. *Am J Kidney Dis* 2002;39:930-6.

[2]   Radovanovic D, Urban P, Simon R, Schmidli M, Maggiorini M, Rickli H, Stauffer JC, Seifert B, Gutzwiller F, Erne P; AMIS Plus Investigators. Outcome of patients with acute coronary syndrome in hospitals of different sizes. A report from the AMIS Plus Registry. *Swiss Med Wkly* 2010;140:314–22.

[3]   Dangas G, Iakovou I, Nikolsky E, Aymong ED, Mintz GS, Kipshidze NN, Lansky AJ, Moussa I, Stone GW, Moses JW, Leon MB, Mehran R. Contrast-induced nephropathy after percutaneous coronary interventions in relation to chronic kidney disease and hemodynamic variables. *Am J Cardiol* 2005;95:13–9.

[4]   Devarajan P. Neutrophil gelatinase-associated lipocalin (NGAL): a new marker of kidney disease. *Scand J Clin Lab Invest Suppl* 2008;241: 89–94.

[5]   Sandler CM. Contrast-agent-induced acute renal dysfunction – is iodixanol the answer? *N Engl J Med* 2003;348:551–3.

[6]   Mehran R, Nikolsky E. Contrast-induced nephropathy: definition, epidemiology, and patients at risk. *Kidney Int Suppl* 2006;100:S11–5.

[7]   ACT Investigators. Acetylcysteine for prevention of renal outcomes in patients undergoing coronary and peripheral vascular angiography: main results from the randomized Acetylcysteine for Contrast-induced nephropathy Trial (ACT). *Circulation* 2011;124:1250–9.

[8] Bolognese L, Falsini G, Schwenke C, Grotti S, Limbruno U, Liistro F, Carrera A, Angioli P, Picchi A, Ducci K, Pierli C. Impact of iso-osmolar versus low-osmolar contrast agents on contrast-induced nephropathy and tissue reperfusion in unselected patients with ST-segment elevation myocardial infarction undergoing primary percutaneous coronary intervention (from the Contrast Media and Nephrotoxicity Following Primary Angioplasty for Acute Myocardial Infarction [CONTRAST-AMI] Trial). *Am J Cardiol* 2012;109:67–74.

[9] Brar SS, Shen AY, Jorgensen MB, Kotlewski A, Aharonian VJ, Desai N, Ree M, Shah AI, Burchette RJ. Sodium bicarbonate vs sodium chloride for the prevention of contrast medium-induced nephropathy in patients undergoing coronary angiography: a randomized trial. *JAMA* 2008;300:1038–46.

[10] Briguori C, Airoldi F, D'Andrea D, Bonizzoni E, Morici N, Focaccio A, Michev I, Montorfano M, Carlino M, Cosgrave J, Ricciardelli B, Colombo A. Renal Insufficiency Following Contrast Media Administration Trial (REMEDIAL): a randomized comparison of 3 preventive strategies. *Circulation* 2007;115:1211–7.

[11] Chen SL, Zhang J, Yei F, Zhu Z, Liu Z, Lin S, Chu J, Yan J, Zhang R, Kwan TW. Clinical outcomes of contrast-induced nephropathy in patients undergoing percutaneous coronary intervention: a prospective, multicenter, randomized study to analyze the effect of hydration and acetylcysteine. *Int J Cardiol* 2008;126:407–13.

[12] Holscher B, Heitmeyer C, Fobker M, Breithardt G, Schaefer RM, Reinecke H. Predictors for contrast media-induced nephropathy and long-term survival: prospectively assessed data from the randomized controlled Dialysis-Versus-Diuresis (DVD) trial. *Can J Cardiol* 2008;24:845–50.

[13] Laskey W, Aspelin P, Davidson C, Rudnick M, Aubry P, Kumar S, Gietzen F, Wiemer M; DXV405 Study Group. Nephrotoxicity of iodixanol versus iopamidol in patients with chronic kidney disease and diabetes mellitus undergoing coronary angiographic procedures. *Am Heart J* 2009;158:822-828.e3.

[14] Lee SW, Kim WJ, Kim YH, Park SW, Park DW, Yun SC, Kim WJ, Suh J, Cho YH, Lee NH, Kang SJ, Lee CW, Park SW, Park SJ. Preventive strategies of renal insufficiency in patients with diabetes undergoing intervention or arteriography (the PREVENT Trial). *Am J Cardiol* 2011;107:1447–52.

[15]   Maioli M, Toso A, Leoncini M, Gallopin M, Tedeschi D, Micheletti C, Bellandi F. Sodium bicarbonate versus saline for the prevention of contrast- induced nephropathy in patients with renal dysfunction undergoing coronary angiography or intervention. *J Am Coll Cardiol* 2008;52:599–604.

[16]   Maioli M, Toso A, Leoncini M, Micheletti C, Bellandi F. Effects of hydration in contrast-induced acute kidney injury after primary angioplasty: a randomized, controlled trial. *Circ Cardiovasc Interv* 2011;4:456–62.

[17]   Morikawa S, Sone T, Tsuboi H, Mukawa H, Morishima I, Uesugi M, Morita Y, Numaguchi Y, Okumura K, Murohara T. Renal protective effects and the prevention of contrast-induced nephropathy by atrial natriuretic peptide. *J Am Coll Cardiol* 2009;53:1040–6.

[18]   Ozcan EE, Guneri S, Akdeniz B, Akyildiz IZ, Senaslan O, Baris N, Asian O, Badak O. Sodium bicarbonate, N-acetylcysteine, and saline for prevention of radiocontrast-induced nephropathy. A comparison of 3 regimens for protecting contrast-induced nephropathy in patients undergoing coronary procedures. A single-center prospective controlled trial. *Am Heart J* 2007;154:539–44.

[19]   Pakfetrat M, Nikoo MH, Malekmakan L, Tabandeh M, RoozbehJ,Nasab MH, Ostovan MA, Salari S, Kafi M, Vaziri NM, Adl F, Hosseini M, Khajehdehi P. A comparison of sodium bicarbonate infusion versus normal saline infusion and its combination with oral acetazolamide for prevention of contrast-induced nephropathy: a randomized, doubleblind trial. *Int Urol Nephrol* 2009;41:629–34.

[20]   Reinecke H, Fobker M, Wellmann J, Becke B, Fleiter J, Heitmeyer C, Breithardt G, Hense HW, Schaefer RM. A randomized controlled trial comparing hydration therapy to additional hemodialysis or N-acetylcysteine for the prevention of contrast medium-induced nephropathy: the Dialysis-versus-Diuresis (DVD) Trial. *Clin Res Cardiol* 2007;96:130–9.

[21]   Rosenstock JL, Bruno R, Kim JK, Lubarsky L, Schaller R, Panagopoulos G, DeVita MV, Michelis MF. The effect of withdrawal of ACE inhibitors or angiotensin receptor blockers prior to coronary angiography on the incidence of contrast-induced nephropathy. *Int Urol Nephrol* 2008;40:749–55.

[22]   Shin DH, Choi DJ, Youn TJ, Yoon CH, Suh JW, Kim KI, Cho YS, Cho GY, Chae IH, Kim CH. Comparison of contrast-induced nephrotoxicity

of iodixanol and iopromide in patients with renal insufficiency undergoing coronary angiography. *Am J Cardiol* 2011;108:189–94.

[23] Solomon RJ, Natarajan MK, Doucet S, Sharma SK, Staniloae CS, Katholi RE, Gelormini JL, Labinaz M, Moreyra AE; Investigators of the CARE Study. Cardiac Angiography in Renally Impaired Patients(CARE) study: a randomized double-blind trial of contrast-induced nephropathy in patients with chronic kidney disease. *Circulation* 2007;115:3189–96.

[24] Thiele H, Hildebrand L, Schirdewahn C, Eitel I, Adams V, Fuernau G, Erbs S, Linke A, Diederich KW, Nowak M, Desch S, Gutberlet M, Schuler G. Impact of high-dose N-acetylcysteine versus placebo on contrastinduced nephropathy and myocardial reperfusion injury in unselected patients with ST-segment elevation myocardial infarction undergoing primary percutaneous coronary intervention. The LIPSIA-N-ACC (Prospective, Single-Blind, Placebo-Controlled, Randomized Leipzig Immediate PercutaneouS Coronary Intervention Acute Myocardial InfarctionN-ACC) Trial. *J Am Coll Cardiol* 2010; 55:2201–9.

[25] Toso A, Maioli M, Leoncini M, Gallopin M, Tedeschi D, Micheletti C,Manzone C, Amato M, Bellandi F. Usefulness of atorvastatin (80 mg) in prevention of contrast-induced nephropathy in patients with chronic renal disease. *Am J Cardiol* 2010;105:288–92.

[26] Wessely R, Koppara T, Bradaric C, Vorpahl M, Braun S, Schulz S, Mehilli J, Schömig A, Kastrati A; Contrast Media and Nephrotoxicity Following Coronary Revascularization by Angioplasty Trial Investigators. Choice of contrast medium in patients with impaired renal function undergoing percutaneous coronary intervention. *Circ Cardiovasc Interv* 2009;2:430–7.

[27] Gruberg L, Mintz GS, Mehran R, Gangas G, Lansky AJ, Kent KM, Pichard AD, Satler LF, Leon MB. The prognostic implications of further renal function deterioration within 48 h of interventional coronary procedures in patients with pre-existent chronic renal insufficiency. *J Am Coll Cardiol* 2000;36:1542-8.

[28] Harjai KJ, Raizada A, Shenoy C, Sattur S, Orshaw P, Yaeger K, Boura J, Aboufares A, Sporn D, Stapleton D. A comparison of contemporary definitions of contrast nephropathy in patients undergoing percutaneous coronary intervention and a proposal for a novel nephropathy grading system. *Am J Cardiol* 2008;101:812-9.

[29] Mehran R, Aymong ED, Nikolsky E, Lasic Z, Iakovou I, Fahy M, Mintz GS, Lansky AJ, Moses JW, Stone GW, Leon MB, Dangas G. A simple risk score for prediction of contrast-induced nephropathy after percutaneous coronary intervention: development and initial validation. *J Am Coll Cardiol* 2004;44:1393–9.

[30] Brown JR, Robb JF, Block CA, Schoolwerth AC, Kaplan AV, O'Connor GT, Solomon RJ, Malenka DJ. Does safe dosing of iodinated contrast prevent contrast-induced acute kidney injury? *Circ Cardiovasc Interv* 2010;3:346–50.

[31] Love L, Johnson MS, Bresler ME, Nelson JE, Olson MC, Flisak ME. The persistent computed tomography nephrogram: its significance in the diagnosis of contrast-associated nephrotoxicity. *Br J Radiol* 1994;67:951–7.

[32] Nickolas TL, Schmidt-Ott KM, Canetta P, Forster C, Singer E, Sise M, Elger A, Maarouf O, Sola-Del Valle DA, O'Rourke M, Sherman E, Lee P, Geara A, Imus P, Guddati A, Polland A, Rahman W, Elitok S, Malik N, Giglio J, El-Sayegh S, Devarajan P, Hebbar S, Saggi SJ, Hahn B, Kettritz R, Luft FC, Barasch J. Diagnostic and prognostic stratification in the emergency department using urinary biomarkers of nephron damage: a multicenter prospective cohort study. *J Am Coll Cardiol* 2012;59:246–55.

[33] Haase M, Devarajan P, Haase-Fielitz A, Bellomo R, Cruz DN, Wagener G, Krawczeski CD, Koyner JL, Murray P, Zappitelli M, Goldstein SL, Makris K, Ronco C, Martensson J, Martling CR, Venge P, Siew E, Ware LB, Ikizler TA, Mertens PR. The outcome of neutrophil gelatinase-associated lipocalin-positive subclinical acute kidney injury: a multicenter pooled analysis of prospective studies. *J Am Coll Cardiol* 2011;57:1752–61.

[34] Alharazy SM, Kong N, Saidin R, Gafor AH, Maskon O, Mohd M, Zakaria SZ. Serum Neutrophil Gelatinase-Associated Lipocalin and Cystatin C are early Biomarkers of Contrast-Induced Nephropathy After Coronary Angiography in Patients With Chronic Kidney Disease. *Angiology* 2013 Apr 11. [Epub ahead of print]

[35] Bachorzewska-Gajewska H, Malyszko J, Sitniewska E, Malyszko JS, Poniatowski B, Pawlak K, Dobrzycki S. NGAL (neutrophil gelatinase-associated lipocalin) and cystatin C: are they good predictors of contrast nephropathy after percutaneous coronary interventions in patients with stable angina and normal serum creatinine? *Int J Cardiol* 2008; 127:290-1.

[36] Shaker OG, El-Shehaby A, El-Khatib M. Early diagnostic markers for contrast nephropathy in patients undergoing coronary angiography. *Angiology* 2010;61:731-6.

[37] Liu XL, Wang ZJ, Yang Q, Yu M, Shen H, Nie B, Han HY, Gao F, Zhou YJ. Plasma neutrophil-gelatinase-associated lipocalin and cystatin C could early diagnose contrast-induced acute kidney injury in patients with renal insufficiency undergoing an elective percutaneous coronary intervention. *Chin Med J (Engl)* 2012;125:1051-6.

[38] Ling W, Zhaohui N, Ben H, Leyi G, Jianping L, Huili D, Jiaqi Q. Urinary IL-18 and NGAL as early predictive biomarkers in contrast-induced nephropathy after coronary angiography. *Nephron Clin Pract* 2008;108:c176-81.

[39] McCullough PA, Williams FJ, Stivers DN, Cannon L, Dixon S, Alexander P, Runyan D, David S. Neutrophil gelatinase-associated lipocalin: a novel marker of contrast nephropathy risk. *Am J Nephrol* 2012;35:509-14.

In: Neutrophil Gelatinase-Associated Lipocalin   ISBN: 978-1-63117-984-6
Editors: M. Hur and S. Di Somma   © 2014 Nova Science Publishers, Inc.

Chapter 17

NGAL in Hypovolemic Patients

*Francesca Orsini[1], Laura Magrini[1], Alan Maisel[2]
and Salvatore Di Somma[1]**
[1]Department of Medical-Surgery Sciences and Translational Medicine,
University Sapienza Rome, Emergency Department Emergency Medicine
Sant'Andrea Hospital, Rome, Italy
[2]Department of Medicine, University of California at San Diego, La Jolla,
CA, US

Abstract

Acute kidney injury (AKI) represents a severe pathological condition common to many critical and potentially life-threatening diseases, such as acute heart failure, sepsis, hypovolemic shock, and contrast-induced nephropathy. NGAL is one of the earliest proteins induced in the kidney after ischemic or nephrotoxic insult. NGAL levels in patients with AKI have been associated with the severity of their prognosis and can be used as a biomarker for AKI. The NGAL level is proportional to the severity of the AKI. Hypovolemia can cause recurrent renal injury. AKI can occur in patients with hypovolemia, if the kidneys do not have enough blood to work. Obtaining NGAL levels in hypovolemic patients may have an impact on clinical outcomes, such us reduction of chronic kidney disease, hospital stay, morbidity, and mortality.

* Correspondence: salvatore.disomma@uniroma1.it.

Introduction

Kidney function is most frequently evaluated by serum creatinine. The fact that creatinine rise is a marker of renal function and not of renal injury makes it less sensitive to early injury that might occur secondary to diuretic treatment or other causes of decreased renal perfusion, such as hypovolemia [1]. NGAL is considered a marker of direct tubular kidney injury since in the cases of AKI, NGAL is secreted in high levels into the blood and urine within 2 hours of acute insult [2].

The pathophysiology of ischemic acute renal failure includes tubular cellular changes (dilated endoplasmic reticulum, clumped nuclear chromatin, swollen mitochondria with small flocculent densities, and the formation of multivesicular bodies). NGAL is one of the earliest proteins secreted by the kidney after ischemic or nephrotoxic insult. NGAL is highly accumulated in the human kidney cortical tubules as well as in the blood and urine after nephrotoxic and ischemic injuries.

Hypovolemia is a critical condition characterized by a decrease of kidney glomerular blood flow. Frequently, without an appropriate and timely treatment, hypovolemia may evolve in hypovolemic shock. Hypovolemic shock is always a medical emergency particularly for the occurrence of acute renal functional damage and needs immediate treatment. Recent studies have demonstrated that NGAL may detect AKI in many critical diseases in the emergency department (ED) and also in the cases of kidney insult due to an acute reduction of glomerular filtration rate that occurs during hypovolemia or hypovolemic shock [3].

AKI is defined as an abrupt deficiency of renal function over a period of hours to days resulting in a failure of the kidney to excrete nitrogenous waste products and to maintain fluid and electrolyte homeostasis. The incidence of AKI is progressively increasing in EDs and the mortality rates of these patients range from 50 to 80% in multiorgan failure. For ED physicians, it is crucial to obtain a rapid diagnosis of AKI, which leads to stop the progressive kidney damage on the basis of an appropriate therapeutic approach [3]. Renal ischemia-reperfusion injury is the leading cause of acute renal injury in native and transplanted kidneys [4]. In current clinical practice, acute renal failure is typically diagnosed by measuring serum creatinine [5].

Unfortunately, creatinine is an unreliable indicator during acute changes in kidney function. Serum creatinine concentrations might not change until about 50% of kidney function has already been lost. Serum creatinine does not accurately depict kidney function until a steady state has been reached, which could take several days [6].

Experimental animal studies have shown that acute renal failure due to ischemia, which is related to acute reduction of glomerular flow, can be prevented only by starting an appropriate and fast restoration of kidney flow, on the basis of fast detection of acute tubular damage [7]. Pathophysiological mechanisms of this type of AKI include diminished renal blood flow, loss of pulsatile flow, hypothermia, atheroembolism, and a generalized inflammatory response [8].

Various clinical algorithms have been proposed for prediction of acute renal failure for these patients, but no methods are available for the early diagnosis of lesser degrees of renal injury. The response of renal tubular cells to an ischemic insult includes cell death; dedifferentiation of viable cells; proliferation, differentiation, and restitution of a normal epithelium. The molecular mechanisms underlying each of these phenomena are under active investigation and hold significant promise for novel therapeutic measures [9].

Hypovolemia

Hypovolemia is defined as the physiological state of reduced blood or, more specifically, reduced plasma volume. When volume loss is severe, homeostatic mechanisms are activated to maintain adequate tissue perfusion to critical organs. These compensatory mechanisms can result in a severe reduction of vascular perfusion and oxygen delivery to numerous other vital organs, such as the liver and the kidneys, which may ultimately lead to multi-organ failure [10].

Absolute hypovolemia means a decrease in the total circulating volume of the blood, which can result from loss of whole blood (external bleeding), loss of plasma (burns), or loss of water from the body resulting in a lower blood volume (severe diarrhea or vomiting, excessive sweating, or urination) [11].

Common causes of hypovolemia include loss of blood (external or internal bleeding or blood donation), loss of plasma (severe burns and lesions discharging fluid), loss of body sodium and consequent intravascular water (excessive sweating, diarrhea, or vomiting), and vasodilation (involving widening of blood vessels, such as trauma, leading to dysfunction of nerve activity on blood vessels; inhibition of the vasomotor center in the brain; or drugs such as vasodilators typically used to treat hypertensive individuals).

Clinical symptoms may not be present until 10 – 20% of total whole-blood volume is lost.

Hypovolemia can be recognized by tachycardia, diminished blood pressure, and the absence of perfusion as assessed by skin signs (skin turning pale) and/or capillary refill on forehead, lips, and nail beds. The patient may feel dizzy, faint, nauseated, or very thirsty. These signs are also characteristic of most types of shock. Hypovolemic shock is an emergency condition, in which severe blood and fluid loss make the heart unable to pump enough blood throughout the body [12].

Hypovolemic shock can cause many organs to stop working, and it is always a medical emergency. However, symptoms and outcomes could be very different. In general, patients with milder degrees of shock tend to do better than those with more severe shock. Severe hypovolemic shock may be fatal, even with immediate medical attention. Generally, elderly patients are more likely to have poor outcomes from shock [13].

An examination may demonstrate classical signs of shock, including: low blood pressure; low body temperature; rapid pulse, often weak and thread. Key steps in the initial management of hypovolemic shock include determining the severity of volume loss, appropriate volume resuscitation, and accurate identification of the underlying cause. The severity of shock can be graded on the basis of the scale of derangement in vital signs, such as heart rate and blood pressure, and by the presence and severity of clinical signs and symptoms, such as pallor, tachypnea, and a reduced level of consciousness. The clinical state of hypovolemic shock can be categorized into three phases: compensated, decompensated, and irreversible. Renal perfusion can be adequately maintained with low to moderate hemorrhages; however, under severe hemorrhage, renal blood flow drops, which cause stimulation of the renin-angiotensin axis and release of angiotensin II, a potent vasoconstrictor and stimulator of aldosterone release [10].

In the context of hypoperfusion and decreased flow to the kidneys, activation of the renin-angiotensin axis leads to dramatic increases in angiotensin II, which results in the constriction of renal efferent arteriole. This part explains the considerable and prolonged cortical hyper-enhancement of the kidneys frequently evaluated by using computed tomography (CT) [14]. Recently, the "black kidney sign," defined as enhancement of the kidneys < 10 HU, has been described in pediatric patients. This extreme hypo-enhancement is an ominous sign and indicates severe hypovolemia [15].

Causes of Hypovolemia

Absolute hypovolemia means a decrease in the volume of the blood, which can result from loss of all blood (external bleeding), loss of plasma (burns), or loss of water from the body resulting in a lower blood volume (severe diarrhea or vomiting, excessive sweating, or urination).

Relative or distributive hypovolemia can occur in the following situations:

- Vasodilation with an increase in the volume of the intravascular space with insufficient blood volume to fill this space and therefore a drop of blood pressure (orthostatic hypotension, vasovagal syncope, neurogenic shock due to spinal cord injury, sepsis, anaphylaxis, side effect of barbiturates and antihypertensives)
- Internal bleeding
- Non-circulating blood within the vascular system (aortic dissection)
- Decreased blood volume in the arteries (arterial hypovolemia) in heart failure
- Decreased oncotic pressure of the blood plasma due to low blood protein levels and hypoalbuminemia (nephrotic syndrome with anasarca, protein malnutrition, ascites — accumulation of the fluid in the abdominal cavity)
- Shift of water from the blood into the body cells (in hyponatremia).

NGAL in Kidney Tubular Cell Damage due to Hypovolemia

As well known, NGAL concentration in the serum and urine has been demonstrated to be a sensitive and specific early marker of AKI after cardiac surgery [16, 17]. It is generally expressed at very low concentrations in several human tissues, including kidney, trachea, lungs, stomach, and colon [18]. NGAL gene is one of the most strikingly upregulated genes (HUGO approved gene name LCN2) and overexpressed in the kidney after ischemia.

In the post-ischemic kidney damage, NGAL is upregulated in several nephron segments, and the protein accumulates predominantly in proximal tubules where it co-localizes with proliferating epithelial cells [19]. NGAL is rapidly induced in kidney tubule cells in response to ischemic injury, and its early appearance in the urine and serum is depending on the amount of reduction in the glomerular filtration rate [17].

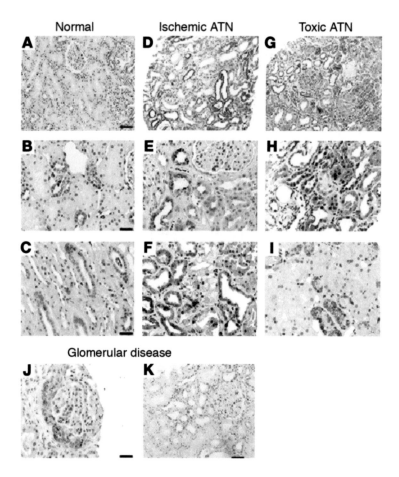

Figure 1. NGAL is expressed in cortical tubules in human acute renal failure. NGAL was detected with affinity-purified polyclonal antibody. (A) The normal kidney had little staining for NGAL. (B and C) At high power, focal staining of distal tubule cells (occupying 10% of the cortical area) and collecting ducts were found. There was no staining of proximal tubules. (D–I) Ischemic acute tubular necrosis (ATN) caused by sepsis (D), by hypovolemia due to vomiting and diarrhea (E), or by heart failure (F), or nephrotoxic ATN caused by bisphosphonate (G), by cephalosporin (H), or by hemoglobinuria (I), produced intense staining of nearly 50% of the cortical tubules. Staining was heterogeneous and most intense in epithelial cells that displayed histologic features of cell injury, including simplification and enlarged reparative nuclei and prominent nucleoli. (J and K). In glomerular diseases, NGAL was weakly expressed by crescents (J) and the proximal tubules of nephrons (K). Scale bars: A, D, G, and K, 11 μm; B, C, E, F, and H–J, 5 μm. *Adapted from Mori et al. [20] with permission.*

NGAL can be expressed in a different way in normal kidneys and in ischemic or toxic kidneys (Figure 1) [20].

Conclusion

NGAL is one of the earliest proteins induced in the kidney after ischemic or nephrotoxic insult. Consequently, NGAL significantly rises in blood and urine soon after AKI [21]. NGAL levels in patients with AKI have been associated with the severity of their prognosis and can be used as a biomarker for AKI. The NGAL level is proportional to the severity of the AKI. Individuals with elevated NGAL levels tend to have higher incidence of renal replacement therapy and have higher rates of in-hospital mortality, both in the presence and the absence of serum creatinine. Therefore, an individual may have AKI without the presence of serum creatinine increase.

The ability to diagnose AKI before acute kidney failure is financially beneficial and favorable for preventive health measures. There is no point of return once there is a significant injury to the kidney; therefore, early diagnosis of kidney injury is important for preventing AKI.

Hypovolemia can cause recurrent renal injury. AKI can occur in patients with hypovolemia, if the kidneys do not have enough blood to work. In conclusion, obtaining NGAL levels in the ED in hypovolemic patients may have an impact on clinical outcomes, such us reduction of chronic kidney disease, hospital stay, morbility, and mortality.

References

[1]   Maisel AS, Mueller C, Fitzgerald R, Brikhan R, Hiestand BC, Iqbal N, Clopton P, van Veldhuisen DJ. Prognostic utility of plasma neutrophil gelatinase-associated lipocalin in patients with acute heart failure: the NGAL evaluation along with b-type natriuretic peptide in acutely decompensated heart failure (GALLANT) trial. *Eur J Heart Fail* 2011;13:846-51.

[2]   Dupont M, Shrestha K, Singh D, Awad A, Kovach C, Scarcipino M, Maroo AP, Tang W. Lack of significant renal tubular injury despite acute kidney injury in acute decompensated heart failure. *Eur J Heart Fail* 2012;14: 597-604.

[3]   Di Somma S, Gori CS, Salvatori E. How to manage cardiorenal syndromes in the emergency room. *Contrib Nephrol* 2010;165:93-100.

[4]   Chen J, Wang W, Zhang Q, Li F, Lei T, Luo D, Zhou H, Yang B. Low molecular weight fucoidan against renal ischemia-reperfusion injury via inhibition of the MAPK signaling pathway. *PLoS One* 2013;8:e56224.

[5]   Devarajan P. Emerging urinary biomarkers in the diagnosis of acute kidney injury. *Expert Opin Med Diagn* 2008; 2: 387–98.

[6]   Dennen P, Parikh CR. Biomarkers of acute kidney injury: can we replace serum creatinine? *Clin Nephrol* 2007;68:269–78.

[7]   Mishra J, Dent C, Tarabishi R, Mitsnefes MM, Ma Q, Kelly C, Ruff SM, Zahedi K, Shao M, Bean J, Mori K, Barasch J, Devarajan P. Neutrophil gelatinase-associated lipocalin (NGAL) as a biomarker for acute renal injury after cardiac surgery. *Lancet* 2005;365:1231-8.

[8]   Devarajan P. Update on mechanisms of ischemic acute kidney injury. *JASN* 2006;17:1503-20.

[9]   Supavekin S, Zhang W, Kucherlapati R, Kaskel FJ, Moore LC, Devarajan P. Differential gene expression following early renal ischemia/reperfusion. *Kidney Int* 2003;63:1714-24.

[10]   Wang J, Liang T, Louis L, Nicolaou S, McLaughlin PD. Hypovolemic shock complex in the trauma setting: a pictorial review. *Can Assoc Radiol J* 2013;64:156-63.

[11]   Kaufman BS, Rackow EC, Falk JL. The relationship between oxygen delivery and consumption during fluid resuscitation of hypovolemic and septic shock. *Chest* 1984;85:336-40.

[12]   Guly HR, Bouamra O, Litte R, Dark P, Coats T, Driscoll P, Lecky FE. Testing the validity of the ATLS classification of hypovolaemic shoek. *Resuscitation* 2010;81:1142-7.

[13]   Bonanno FG. Hemorrhagic shock; the "physiology approach". *J Emerg Trauma Shock* 2012;5:285-95.

[14]   Lubner M, Demertzis J, Lee JY, Appleton CM, Bhalla S, Menias CO. CT evaluation of shock viscera: a pictorial review. *Emerg Radiol* 2008;15;l-11.

[15]   Catalano OA, Napolitano M, Vanzui A. Black kidney sign: a new computed tomographic finding associated with the hypoperfusion complex in children. *J Comput Assist Tomogr* 2005; 29;484-6.

[16]   Krawczeski CD, Woo JG, Wang Y, Michael R, Ma Q, Deverajan P. Neutrophil gelatinase-associated lipocalin concentrations predict development of acute kidney injury in neonates and children after cardiopulmonary bypass. *J Pediatr* 2011;158;1009-15.

[17] Mishra J, Dent C, Tarabishi R,Mitsnefes MM, Ma Q, Kelly C, Ruff SM, Zahedi K, Shao M, Bean J, Mori K, Barasch J, Devarajan P. Neutrophil gelatinase-associated lipocalin (NGAL) as a biomarker for acute renal injury after cardiac surgery. *Lancet* 2005;365:1231-8.

[18] Cowland JB, Borregaard N. Molecular characterization and pattern of tissue expression of the gene for neutrophil gelatinase-associated lipocalin from humans. *Genomics* 1997;45:17–23.

[19] Mishra J, Ma Q, Prada A, Mitsnefes M, Zahedi K, Yang J, Barasch J, Devarajan P. Identification of neutrophil gelatinase-associated lipocalin as a novel urinary biomarker for ischemic injury. *J Am Soc Nephrol* 2003;4:2534–43.

[20] Mori K, Lee HT, Rapoport D, Drexler IR, Foster K, Yang J, Schmidt-Ott KM, Chen X, Li JY, Weiss S, Mishra J, Cheema FH, Markowitz G, Suganami T, Sawai K, Mukoyama M, Kunis C, D'Agati V, Devarajan P, Barasch J. Endocytic delivery of lipocalin-siderophore-iron complex rescues the kidney from ischemia-reperfusion injury. *J Clin Invest* 2005;115:610-21.

[21] Soni SS, Cruz D, Bobek I, Chionh CY, Nalesso F, Lentini P, de Cal M, Corradi V, Virzi G, Ronco C. NGAL: a biomarker of acute kidney injury and other systemic conditions. *Int Urol Nephrol* 2010;42:141-50.

In: Neutrophil Gelatinase-Associated Lipocalin   ISBN: 978-1-63117-984-6
Editors: M. Hur and S. Di Somma   © 2014 Nova Science Publishers, Inc.

Chapter 18

NGAL in Children and Newborns

Laura Magrini[*], *Benedetta De Berardinis*
and Salvatore Di Somma

Department of Medical-Surgery Sciences and Translational Medicine,
University Sapienza Rome, Emergency Department Emergency Medicine
Sant'Andrea Hospital, Rome, Italy

Abstract

Data from the literature show that in children and newborn NGAL
measurement could help in indicating the presence of Acute Kidney
Injury (AKI). Unfortunately little is known about the biomarkers cut-offs
variations in consideration of age and sex, because of the lack of specific
normative ranges of values. In children and newborns, for early detection
of AKI, NGAL has been studied mainly in specific clinical situations
such as cardiopulmonary bypass and sepsis. Results from the current
literature seem to confirm the complementary diagnostic role of NGAL.

Introduction

NGAL participates directly in the development of kidney during
embryonic phases. The promoter region of NGAL gene includes binding site

---
[*] Correspondence: magrinilau@libero.it.

of NF-KB, which controls cell proliferation and survival [1]. It is known that expression of NGAL is elevated in kidney tubular epithelium during the development [2], and it acts as a growth and differentiation factor in multiple cell types, including developing and mature renal epithelia [3]. There are very few data referring to "normal" values of plasma/urinary NGAL in children and newborns. Huynh et al. [4] demonstrated that urinary NGAL levels are correlated with the birth weight; where there seems to be an inverse relationship between NGAL levels and birth weight. In that study, the urinary NGAL was calculated on the basis of body percentiles and demonstrated higher levels and greater variability in females versus males. That study also concluded that a reference range for NGAL in premature infants is similar to that in children and adult. Rybi-Szimińska et al. [5] demonstrated that values of urine NGAL/creatinine ratio were higher in children younger than 6 years of age and systematically decreased with age. In the same cohort of subjects, NGAL was found to be higher in boys than in girls. Cangemi et al. [6] also assessed the urine NGAL in paediatric age and showed that NGAL values in neonates were significantly higher than those in older children. A similar study by Askenazi et al. [7] indicated that urine NGAL declines with chronological age and hypothesized that higher values of urine NGAL in premature children might result from the inability of immature tubules to absorb the protein. However, the interpretation of the results is often quite difficult in paediatric population because of lack of age– and sex–specific normative cut-off values. Previous published urine NGAL values ranged from 1.64 (0.25 – 5.77) ng/mL in healthy children to 5 (2 – 150) ng/mL in very low-birth-weight infants [8, 9].

Sepsis and its related syndromes account for significant morbidity and mortality in critically ill children. Shock and subsequent multiple organ dysfunction remain significant risk factors for mortality in these patients. Sepsis remains a significant risk factor and one of the leading causes of AKI in critically ill children [10]. The risk of late onset sepsis increases with decreasing birth weight and gestational age. On the other hand, the incidence of AKI in the neonatal intensive care unit (NICU) ranges from 8% to 24% with a mortality rate of 10-61%.

There is a growing body of evidence supporting the hypothesis that the sepsis-induced AKI is a separate physiological entity from non septic AKI. First, renal blood flow, both medullar and cortical, is maintained and even increased during severe septic shock. Second, there is an important role for apoptosis, rather than just necrosis, in sepsis and septic shock. Considering these differences, discriminating septic AKI from non–septic AKI may have clinical relevance and prognostic importance. The pathophysiology of sepsis-induced AKI is complex and multifactorial, including intra-renal hemodynamic changes, endothelial dysfunction, infiltration of inflammatory cells in the renal parenchyma, intra-glomerular thrombosis, and obstruction of tubules with necrotic cell and debris. In septic patients, AKI identifies an abrupt decline in kidney function within very few hours after an injury, which leads to functional and structural changes in the kidneys. With the more severe injury, the more likely the overall patient's outcome will be unfavourable. The combination of AKI and sepsis, named sepsis–induced AKI, has been independently associated with an increased risk of death and longer hospital stay [11]. Wheeler et al. [12] showed that there was a significant difference in serum NGAL between healthy children and critically ill children with systemic inflammatory response syndrome. Moreover, in critically ill children with septic shock, NGAL was further increased. Serum NGAL was significantly increased in critically ill children with AKI compared with those without AKI. They concluded that serum NGAL was a highly sensitive predictor of AKI in septic shock children.

In cardiopulmonary bypass (CPB), 2 h after surgery, Mishra et al. [13] demonstrated that the amount of urine NGAL was the most powerful independent predictor of AKI. Another study demonstrated that plasma NGAL, 2 hours (h) after CPB, was the most powerful independent predictor of AKI [14]. The 2 h postoperative plasma NGAL levels strongly correlated with change in creatinine, duration of AKI, and length of hospital stay. Moreover, the 12 h plasma NGAL strongly correlated with mortality. Bennett et al. [15] also showed similar results for urine NGAL. The 2 h urine NGAL levels correlated with severity and duration of AKI, length of hospital stay, dialysis requirement, and death. Krawczeski et al. [16] showed that both plasma and urinary NGAL, when cut-offs were considered, were early predictive biomarkers for AKI and its clinical outcomes after CPB. In neonates, they recommended 2 h plasma NGAL threshold of 100 ng/mL and 2 h urine NGAL threshold of 185 ng/mL for the diagnosis of AKI. Parick et al. [17] showed a good reliability of NGAL not only in diagnosis of AKI after CPB, but also in predicting outcomes. In fact, the first postoperative urine NGAL levels strongly associated with severe AKI. After multivariable adjustment, the highest quintiles of urine IL-18 and urine NGAL of AKI, respectively, compared with the lowest quintiles. Elevated urine NGAL levels were associated with longer hospital stay, longer ICU stay, and duration of mechanical ventilation. The addition of these urine biomarkers improved risk prediction over clinical models alone as measured by net reclassification evaluation and integrated discrimination improvement. In conclusion, among children undergoing cardiac surgery, urine IL-18 and urine NGAL seem to be associated with subsequent AKI and poor outcomes. In a cohort of young patients, Hirsch et al. [18] showed that the administration of iodinated contrast for CPB was associated with both urine and plasma NGAL rise within two hours and the biomarker showed a good sensitivity and specificity in predicting contrast-induced nephropathy.

In a different study, Zappitelli et al. [19] found that urinary NGAL was a useful early marker of AKI in heterogeneous groups of patients (newborns, infants, and children) with unknown timing of kidney injury. In paediatric patients presenting to an emergency department, the accuracy of five putative urinary biomarkers to detect AKI, including urinary NGAL, was very good in predicting patients with pRIFLE Injury versus patients with pRIFLE-Risk or without AKI (Figure 1) [20].

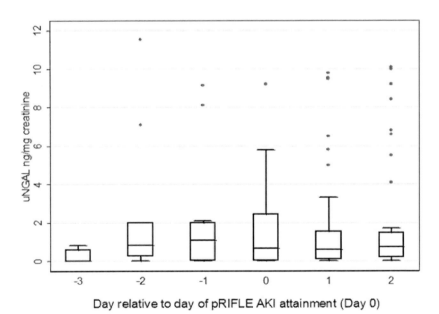

Day relative to day of pRIFLE AKI attainment (Day 0)

Figure 1. uNGAL concentrations from 3 days before to 2 days after sustaining AKI. The center lines represent the median values and the two outer lines represent the interquartile range. Abbreviations: AKI, acute kidney injury; pRIFLE, pediatric modified Risk, Injury, Failure, Loss, End Stage Kidney Disease; uNGAL, urine neutrophil gelatinase-associated lipocalin. *Adapted from Du et al. [20] with permission.*

Conclusion

Similarly to adults, in children and newborns, AKI represents a common and potentially life-threatening problem. In different diseases, NGAL have been demonstrated to be of great utility in detecting AKI in this subset of patients. Although the NGAL cut-off levels are not yet clear, the use of this kidney damage biomarker in children could lead to a decrease in mortality, length of hospital stay, and the use of antibiotic therapy. NGAL could represent a potential, useful biomarker, which is sensitive and specific in different disease processes, in children and newborns.

References

[1]   Häussler U, von Wichert G, Schmid RM, Keller F, Schneider G. Epidermal growth factor activates nuclear factor-kappa B in human proximal tubule cells. *Am J Physiol Renal Physiol* 2005;289:F808-15.

[2]   Mishra J, Mori K, Ma Q, Kelly C, Yang J, Mitsnefes M, Barasch J, Devarajan P. Amelioration of ischemic acute renal injury by neutrophil gelatinase-associated lipocalin. *J Am Soc Nephrol* 2004;15:3073-82.

[3]   Schmidt-Ott KM, Mori K, Li JY, Kalandadze A, Cohen DJ, Devarajan P, Barasch J. Dual action of neutrophil gelatinase-associated lipocalin. *J Am Soc Nephrol* 2007;18:407-13.

[4]   Huynh TK, Bateman DA, Parravicini E, Lorenz JM, Nemerofsky SL, Sise ME, Bowman TM, Polesana E, Barasch JM. Reference values of urinary neutrophil gelatinase-associated lipocalin in very low birth weight infants. *Pediatr Res* 2009;66:528-32.

[5]   Rybi-Szumińska A, Wasilewska A, Litwin M, Kułaga Z, Szumiński M. Paediatric normative data for urine NGAL/creatinine ratio. *Acta Paediatr* 2013;102:e269-72.

[6]   Cangemi G, Storti S, Cantinotti M, Fortunato A, Edmin M, Bruscehttini M, Bugnone D, Melioli G, Clerico A. References values for urinary neuttrophil gelatinase – associated lipocalin (NGAL) in pediatric age measured with a fully automated chemiluminescent platform. *Clin Chem Lab Med* 2012; 51: 1101–5.

[7]   Askenazi DJ, Koralkar R, Levitan EB, Goldstein SL, Devarajan P, Khandrika S, Mehta RL, Ambalavanan N. Baseline values of candidate

urine acute kidney injury biomarkers vary by gestational age in premature infants. *Pediatr Res* 2011;70:302-6.

[8]   Wasilewska A, Taranta-Janusz K, Dębek W, Zoch-Zwierz W, Kuroczycka-Saniutycz E. KIM-1 and NGAL: new markers of obstructive nephropathy. *Pediatr Nephrol* 2011;26:579-86.

[9]   Huynh TK, Bateman DA, Parravicini E, Lorenz JM, Nemerofsky SL, Sise ME, Bowman TM, Polesana E, Barasch JM. Reference values of urinary neutrophil gelatinase-associated lipocalin in very low birth weight infants. *Pediatr Res* 2009;66:528-32.

[10]   Wheeler DS, Devarajan P, Ma Q, Harmon K, Monaco M, Cvijanovich N, Wong HR. Serum neutrophil gelatinase-associated lipocalin (NGAL) as a marker of acute kidney injury in critically ill children with septic shock. *Crit Care Med* 2008;36:1297-303.

[11]   Mussap M, Noto A, Fravega M, Fanos V. Urine neutrophil gelatinase-associated lipocalin (uNGAL) and netrin-1: are they effectively improving the clinical management of sepsis-induced acute kidney injury (AKI)? *J Matern Fetal Neonatal Med* 2011;S2:15-7.

[12]   Wheeler DS, Devarajan P, Ma Q, Harmon K, Monaco M, Cvijanovich N, Wong HR. Serum neutrophil gelatinase-associated lipocalin (NGAL) as a marker of acute kidney injury in critically ill children with septic shock. *Crit Care Med* 2008;36:1297-303.

[13]   Mishra J, Dent C, Tarabishi R, Mitsnefes MM, Ma Q, Kelly C, Ruff SM, Zahedi K, Shao M, Bean J, Mori K, Barasch J, Devarajan P. Neutrophil gelatinase-associated lipocalin (NGAL) as a biomarker for acute renal injury after cardiac surgery. *Lancet* 2005;365:1231-8.

[14]   Dent CL, Ma Q, Dastrala S, Bennett M, Mitsnefes MM, Barasch J, Devarajan P. Plasma neutrophil gelatinase-associated lipocalin predicts acute kidney injury, morbidity and mortality after pediatric cardiac surgery: a prospective uncontrolled cohort study. *Crit Care* 2007;11:R127.

[15]   Bennett M, Dent CL, Ma Q, Dastrala S, Grenier F, Workman R, Syed H, Ali S, Barasch J, Devarajan P. Urine NGAL predicts severity of acute kidney injury after cardiac surgery: a prospective study. *Clin J Am Soc Nephrol* 2008;3:665-73.

[16]   Krawczeski CD, Woo JG, Wang Y, Bennett MR, Ma Q, Devarajan P. Neutrophil gelatinase-associated lipocalin concentrations predict development of acute kidney injury in neonates and children after cardiopulmonary bypass. *J Pediatr* 2011;158:1009-1015.

[17] Parikh CR, Devarajan P, Zappitelli M, Sint K, Thiessen-Philbrook H, Li S, Kim RW, Koyner JL, Coca SG, Edelstein CL, Shlipak MG, Garg AX, Krawczeski CD; TRIBE-AKI Consortium. Postoperative biomarkers predict acute kidney injury and poor outcomes after pediatric cardiac surgery. *J Am Soc Nephrol* 2011;22:1737-47.

[18] Hirsch R, Dent C, Pfriem H, Allen J, Beekman RH 3rd, Ma Q, Dastrala S, Bennett M, Mitsnefes M, Devarajan P. NGAL is an early predictive biomarker of contrast-induced nephropathy in children. *Pediatr Nephrol* 2007;22:2089-95.

[19] Zappitelli M, Washburn KK, Arikan AA, Loftis L, Ma Q, Devarajan P, Parikh CR, Goldstein SL. Urine neutrophil gelatinase-associated lipocalin is an early marker of acute kidney injury in critically ill children: a prospective cohort study. *Crit Care* 2007;11:R84.

[20] Du Y, Zappitelli M, Mian A, Bennett M, Ma Q, Devarajan P, Mehta R, Goldstein SL. Urinary biomarkers to detect acute kidney injury in the pediatric emergency center. *Pediatr Nephrol* 2011;26:267-74.

In: Neutrophil Gelatinase-Associated Lipocalin   ISBN: 978-1-63117-984-6
Editors: M. Hur and S. Di Somma   © 2014 Nova Science Publishers, Inc.

Chapter 19

NGAL as Marker for Prognosis of Acute Kidney Injury

Michael Haase [*] *and Anja Haase-Fielitz*

Department of Nephrology, Hypertension, Diabetes and Endocrinology,
Otto-von-Guericke University Magdeburg, Germany

Abstract

Prognosis of a disease has a central role in clinical decision-making. A *prognostic biomarker* is a marker that provides information on the likely course and outcome of the disease. In a genomwide screening for novel renal biomarkers and proteomic follow-up experiments, neutrophil gelatinase-associated lipocalin (NGAL) was identified as the gene with the highest mRNA and protein levels in the kidney, urine, and plasma and with the earliest rise and peak after renal ischemia. The observed dose-effect response in numerous animal and human studies makes a favorable prognostic value for NGAL likely. The prognostic value of NGAL has now been investigated in several thousands of patients undergoing cardiac surgery, kidney transplantation, or critical illness. Five years after the initial meta-analysis, the overall value of NGAL for prognosis of acute kidney injury (AKI) and associated adverse outcomes across various patient populations remains essentially unchanged. The most frequently reported endpoints in biomarker studies on AKI prognosis are:

[*] Correspondence: michael.haase@med.ovgu.de.

AKI progression, requirement of renal replacement therapy (RRT), transition of AKI to chronic kidney disease (CKD), and mortality. This chapter condenses recent data on NGAL as marker for AKI prognosis.

Introduction

Numerous studies indicate that onset of acute kidney injury (AKI) is associated with a higher resource utilization and adverse events compared to patients without AKI [1, 2]. Prognosis of a disease has a central role in clinical decision-making. A *prognostic biomarker* is a marker that provides information on the likely course and outcome of the disease. Transferred to AKI, this refers to the probability of an affected patient developing acute or chronic renal complications over a specific period of time.

Of note, patients who recover from AKI often do not differ in major clinical characteristics from those patients who do not recover [3]. The need for novel biomarkers to permit earlier diagnosis of AKI but also to provide early information on the *prognosis* and the underlying pathophysiology is therefore well acknowledged. Accordingly, such markers may help identify patients with likely failure to recover back to baseline renal function after an episode of AKI.

Which options do we have at present to complement clinical data and classical routine measures such as ultrasound with molecular information on the course of kidney disease? The type and the extent of tissue damage inform the prognosis of renal disease, but kidney biopsy is not a routine test. Biochemical tests that correlate with specific histological findings might serve as surrogates for the kidney biopsy. In this regard, renal tubular damage has recently been recognized to be a major and early pathophysiological event, which occurs prior to acute changes in renal function. In current clinical practice, however, the concept and diagnosis of AKI are mainly based on changes in renal excretion function using serum creatinine and urinary output. Diagnosis of AKI using creatinine- and urinary output-based RIFLE [4], AKI Network [5], or KDIGO consensus criteria [6] is of prognostic relevance [7 - 9]. However, such a diagnosis is delayed by 24 - 72 hours compared to the diagnosis by means of novel renal biomarkers indicating tubular damage such as neutrophil gelatinase-associated lipocalin (NGAL) [10 - 12]. Kidney epithelia express and excrete substantial quantities of NGAL, a siderophore-iron-binding protein, when damaged by diverse etiologic insults [13]. NGAL regulates intrarenal iron metabolism and acts to stimulate proliferation and epithelialization. A single systemic administration of the iron-transporting form of NGAL protects the kidney and mitigates renal injury [14, 15]. It has been speculated that the increase in the NGAL level after renal tubular injury may serve to limit injury in recurrent insults or ameliorate the degree of damage in an ongoing insult, both pointing toward a biological role of NGAL for AKI prognosis.

Tubular damage markers may add valuable information for prognosis of AKI and associated complications with regard to i) earlier assessment of a prognosis compared to routine biological markers of renal function, and ii) identification of a previously undetected group of patients with kidney injury but without acute loss of renal function.

Translating these requirements to a valuable prognostic-relevant renal biomarker, such markers would need to inform about i) AKI progression and severity; ii) basing on AKI-to- chronic kidney disease (CKD) transition, the development or worsening of CKD; iii) requirement of acute and/or chronic renal replacement therapy (RRT); iv) hospital- or long-term mortality; and v) length of hospitalization (*Figure 1*).

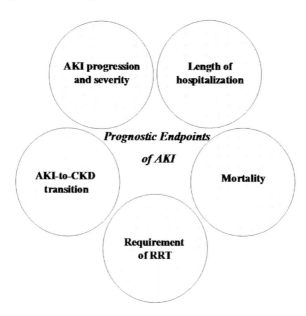

Figure 1. Clinical endpoints reported in studies using renal biomarkers for prognosis. AKI, acute kidney injury; CKD, chronic kidney disease; RRT, renal replacement therapy.

Main Findings

AKI Progression and Severity

Clinicians have limited tools to determine which patients will progress to more severe or prolonged forms of AKI. In a study with a focus on AKI progression enrolling 161 hospitalized patients with established AKI, NGAL independently predicted the composite endpoint that included progression to a higher RIFLE-AKI class, dialysis, or death when corrected for demographics, comorbidities, creatinine, and AKI severity [16]. Plasma NGAL measured on the day of AKI diagnosis in patients after cardiac surgery improved risk stratification for worsening AKI stage according to AKIN criteria [5] compared with the clinical model alone (category-free net reclassification improvement of 0.69, $P < 0.0001$) [17]. Measurement of urine NGAL 6 hours after elective coronary procedure predicted the severity of contrast-induced AKI according to recent KDIGO consensus criteria [6] in patients with pre-existing CKD [18].

Several studies demonstrate that the prognostic value of NGAL seems to increase with severity of acute renal function loss [11, 19]. This was confirmed in a recent study enrolling a cohort of 95 patients with AKIN stage 1, where NGAL predicted worsening of AKI or mortality with an area under the receiver operating characteristic curve (AUC) of 0.72 and the progression to AKIN stage 3 or mortality with an AUC of 0.83 [20]. These studies support the view that, as all currently used AKI definitions are based on changes in serum creatinine and urine output, they may not at all reflect the true value of NGAL in detecting AKI but rather the limitations of current surrogates for the presence or absence of AKI.

In other words, a biomarker can only be as good as the surrogate endpoint it predicts—in the case of NGAL, serum creatinine- and urine output-based AKI, insensitive or unspecific markers of loss of GFR, respectively [19]. In a 'Gedankenexperiment', Waikar et al. [21] proved this point generating statistics on the following example: if AKI incidence is 40%, and the biochemical gold standard for AKI diagnosis (serum creatinine) has an assumed sensitivity of 80% and specificity of 80% for 'true' AKI, even a 'perfect' tubular damage biomarker (100% sensitive, 100% specific) for 'true' AKI will yield in a clinical study a sensitivity of 50% and a specificity of 94% for predicting an imperfect gold standard, which is creatinine-based AKI (not the disease).

In a cohort of 100 adult cardiac surgery patients, Haase *et al.* [22] found that NGAL correlated with and was independent predictor of AKI severity as evidenced by AKI duration and AKI grade after adult cardiac surgery; findings which were in line with those reported in a pediatric population also undergoing cardiac surgery [23]. In the latter study, urine NGAL measured 2 hours after start of cardiopulmonary bypass (CPB) using ARCHITECT assay correlated with grade and duration of AKI, length of stay, dialysis requirement, and death [23].

Preliminary Evidence for Role of NGAL in AKI-to-CKD Transition

After damage, the kidney has the ability to repair itself to a certain degree. With mild injury, this repair may be performed *ad integrum* and become indistinguishable from healthy tissue. However, when acute tissue damage is more severe or superimposed on pre-existing kidney impairment, the repair process may lead to (partial) organ fibrosis, which may be the first step towards CKD. Thus, AKI may not represent a fully benign event and rather set the stage for chronic disease with structural alterations of the kidney tissue architecture [24, 25].

Preliminary data generated from experimental ischemia-reperfusion injury models in mice demonstrated sustained upregulation of KIM-1- and NGAL-genes during the kidney repair phase associated with impaired regulation of cell cycle and chemotaxis, which contributed to progressive renal fibrosis [26]. Persistent immune and inflammatory responses during the repair phase might explain progressive renal injury after ischemia-reperfusion. Mechanistic evidence grows for a causal link of AKI with the *de novo* development or progression of CKD [27, 28], which has also been supported by epidemiological studies [29]. Even "apparently" full kidney recovery confers an increased risk for subsequent development of CKD [30].

While in theory, NGAL may be a good predictor of AKI-to-CKD-transition, study data are sparse. The only clinical study so far in the biomarker field reported that in patients with acute-on-chronic kidney injury, urinary NGAL level correlated with the severity of AKI on CKD, while urinary α1-microglobulin expression correlated with the degree of renal function recovery [31].

Renal Recovery

Rapid resolution of AKI might be a good prognostic indicator. Being able to predict whether AKI will resolve could improve patient monitoring and care. There are first data on sufficient value of NGAL indicating renal recovery [32, 33]. In the first study, recovery was defined as alive and not requiring RRT during hospitalization or having a persistent RIFLE-F classification at hospital discharge. The reclassification of risk of renal recovery in patients with community-acquired pneumonia significantly improved by 17%, when NGAL was combined with the clinical model that included age, serum creatinine, pneumonia severity, and nonrenal organ failure [32]. However, another study available to date reported NGAL to be a poor predictor for renal recovery following AKI after major surgery [33].

Requirement of Renal Replacement Therapy

Given the limitations of serum creatinine and urine output, alternative renal endpoints have been proposed. Knowledge on the likelihood of initiation of RRT may influence clinical decision-making. On the other hand, evaluation of the requirement of RRT as a renal endpoint for biomarker studies seems to be highly variable. Timing of RRT initiation varies according to i) individual case-specific dynamics of renal function deterioration; ii) logistic circumstances which may differ from country to country and hospital to hospital; and iii) clinical risk assessment, even from physician to physician.

In 2009, a meta-analysis reported on the value of NGAL pooling data from 1,948 patients with 84 of those requiring RRT [34]. An AUC was 0.78 and, at a cut-off value of > 278 ng/mL, sensitivity was 76% and specificity 80%. The risk of patients with NGAL concentration above cut-off was 13 times higher for RRT compared to those patients presenting with NGAL concentration below cut-off [34]. Several studies added more information to these numbers. In these more recent studies, average AUCs for RRT prediction were similar to previous results of the meta-analysis [11, 35 - 40]. Also, in neonates and infants with AKI, NGAL seems to be a valuable predictive tool of RRT requirement with number needed to screen to correctly identify the risk of RRT or death in one patient between 1.5 and 2.6 within 12 hours postoperatively [41]. However, NGAL cut-off values reported for RRT varied up to > 1,000 ng/mL [42]. A minority of studies reported NGAL not being valuable for RRT prediction [43].

Acute tubular damage may occur without detectable loss of excretory function and *vice versa* and may predict worse clinical outcome with NGAL and serum creatinine reflecting distinct pathophysiological events [44]. The concept of outcomes in "biomarker-positive, creatinine-negative" patients has recently been explored as exemplary demonstrated in *Figure 2* [44 - 46]. There are three studies enrolling about 4,500 cardiac surgical, critically ill, or emergency department patients who were grouped according to their NGAL and serum creatinine status (NGAL-/sCrea-, NGAL+/sCrea-, NGAL-/sCrea+, NGAL+/sCrea+). These studies found that measurement of the levels of NGAL complemented the information obtained by measurement of serum creatinine levels in establishing the diagnosis of AKI and predicting prognosis. A substantial proportion of patients (15 – 20%) had elevated NGAL levels even in the absence of a rise in serum creatinine. This previously undetectable condition ("subclinical AKI") was associated with a 2–3-fold increased risk of death or the need for RRT compared to that of patients in whom serum creatinine was not elevated. Notably, even in patients with significant loss of renal function, measurement of tubule damage biomarker levels still added prognostic information, as patients with increased levels of both NGAL and serum creatinine levels displayed by far the worst prognosis [47].

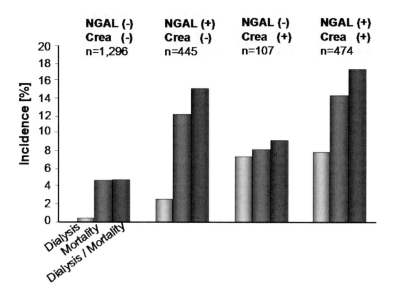

Figure 2. NGAL-detected acute tubular damage associates with poor prognosis. NGAL, neutrophil gelatinase-associated lipocalin; crea, creatinine.

Mortality

The aforementioned NGAL meta-analysis [34] reported a somewhat lower value for NGAL predicting mortality (AUC 0.71) compared to predicting AKI or RRT requirement. Such a modest performance below AKI predictive value has been confirmed by several more recent studies [11, 46]. These results may reflect that mortality may not solely be associated with renal complications, with the latter potentially being correctly identified by NGAL. However, as a component of multivariate analyses, addition of NGAL improved prediction of mortality [11, 12, 39, 40]. Finally, when measured at inception of RRT, NGAL predicted survival in critically ill patients with AKI [48].

Length of Hospitalization

Although duration of hospitalization has been reported in many of kidney biomarker studies, such an endpoint is influenced from too many non-renal and at times more logistical than medical constraints. Also, external validity of duration of hospital stay is limited given differences between health care providers and organization but also between countries. Nonetheless, studies reporting on this endpoint found a clear correlation between NGAL concentration in urine or plasma and length of hospitalization [22, 23].

Conclusion

NGAL seems to have a sufficient prognostic value for diverse endpoints after AKI. Clinical implementation of NGAL will depend on availability of laboratory platforms and readiness of physicians to include NGAL test result in their clinical decision-making process.

References

[1]   Uchino S, Kellum JA, Bellomo R, Doig GS, Morimatsu H, Morgera S, Schetz M, Tan I, Bouman C, Macedo E, Gibney N, Tolwani A, Ronco C; Beginning and Ending Supportive Therapy for the Kidney (BEST

Kidney) Investigators. Acute renal failure in critically ill patients: a multinational, multicenter study. *JAMA* 2005;294:813–18.

[2] Hoste EA, Clermont G, Kersten A, Venkataraman R, Angus DC, De Bacquer D, Kellum JA. RIFLE criteria for acute kidney injury are associated with hospital mortality in critically ill patients: a cohort analysis. *Crit. Care* 2006;10:R73.

[3] Bhandari S, Turney JH. Survivors of acute renal failure who do not recover renal function. *QJM* 1996;89:415-21.

[4] Bellomo R, Ronco C, Kellum JA, Mehta RL, Palevsky P, Acute Dialysis Quality Initiative workgroup; Acute renal failure - definition, outcome measures, animal models, fluid therapy and information technology needs: the Second International Consensus Conference of the Acute Dialysis Quality Initiative (ADQI) Group. *Crit. Care* 2004;8:R204-12.

[5] Mehta RL, Kellum JA, Shah SV, Molitoris BA, Ronco C, Warnock DG, Levin A; Acute Kidney Injury Network. Acute Kidney Injury Network: report of an initiative to improve outcomes in acute kidney injury. *Crit. Care* 2007;11:R31.

[6] KDIGO Clinical Practice Guideline for Acute Kidney Injury. Kidney Int Suppl 2012 doi:10.1038/kisup.2012

[7] Uchino S, Bellomo R, Goldsmith D, Bates S, Ronco C. An assessment of the RIFLE criteria for acute renal failure in hospitalized patients. *Crit. Care Med.* 2006;34:1913-7.

[8] Shinjo H, Sato W, Imai E. Comparison of Kidney Disease: Improving Global Outcomes and Acute Kidney Injury Network criteria for assessing patients in intensive care units. *Clin. Exp. Nephrol.* 2013 Nov 27. [Epub ahead of print]

[9] Zeng X, McMahon GM, Brunelli SM, Bates DW, Waikar SS. Incidence, Outcomes, and Comparisons across Definitions of AKI in Hospitalized Individuals. *Clin. J. Am. Soc. Nephrol.* 2014;9:12-20.

[10] Haase-Fielitz A, Bellomo R, Devarajan P, Story D, Matalanis G, Dragun D, Haase M. Novel and conventional serum biomarkers predicting acute kidney injury in adult cardiac surgery-a prospective cohort study. *Crit. Care Med.* 2009;37:553-60.

[11] de Geus HR, Bakker J, Lesaffre EM, le Noble JL. Neutrophil gelatinase-associated lipocalin at ICU admission predicts for acute kidney injury in adult patients. *Am. J. Respir. Crit. Care Med.* 2011;183:907-14.

[12] Shapiro NI, Trzeciak S, Hollander JE, Birkhahn R, Otero R, Osborn TM, Moretti E, Nguyen HB, Gunnerson K, Milzman D, Gaieski DF, Goyal M, Cairns CB, Kupfer K, Lee SW, Rivers EP. The diagnostic accuracy

of plasma neutrophil gelatinase-associated lipocalin in the prediction of acute kidney injury in emergency department patients with suspected sepsis. *Ann. Emerg. Med.* 2010;56:52-59.

[13] Haase M, Bellomo R, Haase-Fielitz A. Neutrophil gelatinase-associated lipocalin. *Curr. Opin. Crit. Care* 2010;16:526-32.

[14] Mori K, Lee HT, Rapoport D, Drexler IR, Foster K, Yang J, Schmidt-Ott KM, Chen X, Li JY, Weiss S, Mishra J, Cheema FH, Markowitz G, Suganami T, Sawai K, Mukoyama M, Kunis C, D'Agati V, Devarajan P, Barasch J. Endocytic delivery of lipocalin-siderophore-iron complex rescues the kidney from ischemia-reperfusion injury. *J. Clin. Invest.* 2005;115:610-21.

[15] Mishra J, Mori K, Ma Q, Kelly C, Yang J, Mitsnefes M, Barasch J, Devarajan P. Amelioration of ischemic acute renal injury by neutrophil gelatinase-associated lipocalin. *J. Am. Soc. Nephrol.* 2004;15:3073-82.

[16] Singer E, Elger A, Elitok S, Kettritz R, Nickolas TL, Barasch J, Luft FC, Schmidt-Ott KM. Urinary neutrophil gelatinase-associated lipocalin distinguishes pre-renal from intrinsic renal failure and predicts outcomes. *Kidney Int.* 2011;80:405-14.

[17] Koyner JL, Garg AX, Coca SG, Sint K, Thiessen-Philbrook H, Patel UD, Shlipak MG, Parikh CR; TRIBE-AKI Consortium. Biomarkers predict progression of acute kidney injury after cardiac surgery. *J. Am. Soc. Nephrol.* 2012;23:905-14.

[18] Tasanarong A, Hutayanon P, Piyayotai D. Urinary Neutrophil Gelatinase-Associated Lipocalin predicts the severity of contrast-induced acute kidney injury in chronic kidney disease patients undergoing elective coronary procedures. *BMC Nephrol.* 2013;14:270.

[19] Haase-Fielitz A, Bellomo R, Devarajan P, Bennett M, Story D, Matalanis G, Frei U, Dragun D, Haase M. The predictive performance of plasma neutrophil gelatinase-associated lipocalin (NGAL) increases with grade of acute kidney injury. *Nephrol. Dial. Transplant.* 2009;24:3349-54.

[20] Arthur JM, Hill EG, Alge JL, Lewis EC, Neely BA, Janech MG, Tumlin JA, Chawla LS, Shaw AD. Evaluation of 32 urine biomarkers to predict the progression of acute kidney injury after cardiac surgery. *Kidney Int.* 2013 Sep 4. doi: 10.1038/ki.2013.333. [Epub ahead of print]

[21] Waikar SS, Betensky RA, Emerson SC, Bonventre JV. Imperfect gold standards for kidney injury biomarker evaluation. *J. Am. Soc. Nephrol.* 2012;23:13-21.

[22] Haase M, Bellomo R, Devarajan P, Ma Q, Bennett MR, Möckel M, Matalanis G, Dragun D, Haase-Fielitz A. Novel biomarkers early predict the severity of acute kidney injury after cardiac surgery in adults. *Ann. Thorac. Surg.* 2009;88:124-30.

[23] Bennett M, Dent CL, Ma Q, Dastrala S, Grenier F, Workman R, Syed H, Ali S, Barasch J, Devarajan P. Urine NGAL predicts severity of acute kidney injury after cardiac surgery: a prospective study. *Clin. J. Am. Soc. Nephrol.* 2008;3:665-73.

[24] Coca SG. Is it AKI or nonrecovery of renal function that is important for long-term outcomes? *Clin. J. Am. Soc. Nephrol.* 2012;8:173-176.

[25] Coca SG, Garg AX, Thiessen-Philbrook H, Koyner JL, Patel UD, Krumholz HM, Shlipak MG, Parikh CR; for the TRIBE-AKI Consortium. Urinary Biomarkers of AKI and Mortality 3 Years after Cardiac Surgery. *J. Am. Soc. Nephrol.* 2013 Dec 19. [Epub ahead of print].

[26] Ko GJ, Grigoryev DN, Linfert D, Jang HR, Watkins T, Cheadle C, Racusen L, Rabb H. Transcriptional analysis of kidneys during repair from AKI reveals possible roles for NGAL and KIM-1 as biomarkers of AKI-to-CKD transition. *Am. J. Physiol. Renal. Physiol.* 2010; 298:F1472-83.

[27] Yang L, Besschetnova TY, Brooks CR, Shah JV, Bonventre JV. Epithelial cell cycle arrest in G2/M mediates kidney fibrosis after injury. *Nat. Med.* 2010;16:535-43.

[28] Humphreys BD, Xu F, Sabbisetti V, Grgic I, Naini SM, Wang N, Chen G, Xiao S, Patel D, Henderson JM, Ichimura T, Mou S, Soeung S, McMahon AP, Kuchroo VK, Bonventre JV. Chronic epithelial kidney injury molecule-1 expression causes murine kidney fibrosis. *J. Clin. Invest.* 2013;123:4023-35.

[29] Ishani A, Xue JL, Himmelfarb J, Eggers PW, Kimmel PL, Molitoris BA, Collins AJ. Acute kidney injury increases risk of ESRD among elderly. *J. Am. Soc. Nephrol.* 2009;20:223-8.

[30] Bucaloiu ID, Kirchner HL, Norfolk ER, Hartle JE 2nd, Perkins RM. Increased risk of death and de novo chronic kidney disease following reversible acute kidney injury. Kidney Int 2012;81:477-85.

[31] Luk CC, Chow KM, Kwok JS, Kwan BC, Chan MH, Lai KB, Lai FM, Wang G, Li PK, Szeto CC. Urinary biomarkers for the prediction of reversibility in acute-on-chronic renal failure. *Dis. Markers* 2013;34:179-85.

[32] Srisawat N, Murugan R, Lee M, Kong L, Carter M, Angus DC, Kellum JA; Genetic and Inflammatory Markers of Sepsis (GenIMS) Study Investigators. Plasma neutrophil gelatinase-associated lipocalin predicts recovery from acute kidney injury following community-acquired pneumonia. *Kidney Int.* 2011;80:545-52.

[33] Zeng XF, Li JM, Tan Y, Wang ZF, He Y, Chang J, Zhang H, Zhao H, Bai X, Xie F, Sun J, Zhang Y. Performance of urinary NGAL and L-FABP in predicting acute kidney injury and subsequent renal recovery: a cohort study based on major surgeries. *Clin. Chem. Lab. Med.* 2013 Nov 29:1-8. doi: 10.1515/cclm-2013-0823. [Epub ahead of print]

[34] Haase M, Bellomo R, Devarajan P, Schlattmann P, Haase-Fielitz A; NGAL Meta-analysis Investigator Group. Accuracy of neutrophil gelatinase-associated lipocalin (NGAL) in diagnosis and prognosis in acute kidney injury: a systematic review and meta-analysis. *Am. J. Kidney Dis.* 2009;54:1012-24.

[35] Endre ZH, Pickering JW, Walker RJ, Devarajan P, Edelstein CL, Bonventre JV, Frampton CM, Bennett MR, Ma Q, Sabbisetti VS, Vaidya VS, Walcher AM, Shaw GM, Henderson SJ, Nejat M, Schollum JB, George PM. Improved performance of urinary biomarkers of acute kidney injury in the critically ill by stratification for injury duration and baseline renal function. *Kidney Int.* 2011;79:1119-30.

[36] Camou F, Oger S, Paroissin C, Guilhon E, Guisset O, Mourissoux G, Pouyes H, Lalanne T, Gabinski C. Plasma Neutrophil Gelatinase-Associated Lipocalin (NGAL) predicts acute kidney injury in septic shock at ICU admission. *Ann. Fr. Anesth. Reanim.* 2013;32:157-64.

[37] Valette X, Savary B, Nowoczyn M, Daubin C, Pottier V, Terzi N, Seguin A, Fradin S, Charbonneau P, Hanouz JL, du Cheyron D. Accuracy of plasma neutrophil gelatinase-associated lipocalin in the early diagnosis of contrast-induced acute kidney injury in critical illness. *Intensive Care Med.* 2013;39:857-65.

[38] Siew ED, Ware LB, Bian A, Shintani A, Eden SK, Wickersham N, Cripps B, Ikizler TA. Distinct injury markers for the early detection and prognosis of incident acute kidney injury in critically ill adults with preserved kidney function. *Kidney Int.* 2013;84:786-94.

[39] Parikh CR, Devarajan P, Zappitelli M, Sint K, Thiessen-Philbrook H, Li S, Kim RW, Koyner JL, Coca SG, Edelstein CL, Shlipak MG, Garg AX, Krawczeski CD; TRIBE-AKI Consortium. Postoperative biomarkers predict acute kidney injury and poor outcomes after pediatric cardiac surgery. *J. Am. Soc. Nephrol.* 2011;22:1737-47.

[40] Parikh CR, Coca SG, Thiessen-Philbrook H, Shlipak MG, Koyner JL, Wang Z, Edelstein CL, Devarajan P, Patel UD, Zappitelli M, Krawczeski CD, Passik CS, Swaminathan M, Garg AX; TRIBE-AKI Consortium. Postoperative biomarkers predict acute kidney injury and poor outcomes after adult cardiac surgery. *J. Am. Soc. Nephrol.* 2011;22:1748-57.

[41] Bojan M, Vicca S, Lopez-Lopez V, Mogenet A, Pouard P, Falissard B, Journois D. Predictive Performance of Urine Neutrophil Gelatinase-Associated Lipocalin for Dialysis Requirement and Death Following Cardiac Surgery in Neonates and Infants. *Clin. J. Am. Soc. Nephrol.* 2013 Nov 21. [Epub ahead of print]

[42] Tiranathanagul K, Amornsuntorn S, Avihingsanon Y, Srisawat N, Susantitaphong P, Praditpornsilpa K, Tungsanga K, Eiam-Ong S. Potential role of neutrophil gelatinase-associated lipocalin in identifying critically ill patients with acute kidney injury stage 2-3 who subsequently require renal replacement therapy. *Ther. Apher. Dial.* 2013;17:332-8.

[43] Royakkers AA, Bouman CS, Stassen PM, Korevaar JC, Binnekade JM, van de Hoek W, Kuiper MA, Spronk PE, Schultz MJ. Systemic and urinary neutrophil gelatinase-associated lipocalins are poor predictors of acute kidney injury in unselected critically ill patients. *Crit. Care Res. Pract.* 2012;2012:712695.

[44] Haase M, Devarajan P, Haase-Fielitz A, Bellomo R, Cruz DN, Wagener G, Krawczeski CD, Koyner JL, Murray P, Zappitelli M, Goldstein SL, Makris K, Ronco C, Martensson J, Martling CR, Venge P, Siew E, Ware LB, Ikizler TA, Mertens PR. The outcome of neutrophil gelatinase-associated lipocalin-positive subclinical acute kidney injury: a multicenter pooled analysis of prospective studies. *J. Am. Coll. Cardiol.* 2011 26;57:1752-61.

[45] Nickolas TL, Schmidt-Ott KM, Canetta P, Forster C, Singer E, Sise M, Elger A, Maarouf O, Sola-Del Valle DA, O'Rourke M, Sherman E, Lee P, Geara A, Imus P, Guddati A, Polland A, Rahman W, Elitok S, Malik N, Giglio J, El-Sayegh S, Devarajan P, Hebbar S, Saggi SJ, Hahn B, Kettritz R, Luft FC, Barasch J. Diagnostic and prognostic stratification in the emergency department using urinary biomarkers of nephron damage: a multicenter prospective cohort study. *J. Am. Coll. Cardiol.* 2012;59:246-55.

[46] Di Somma S, Magrini L, De Berardinis B, Marino R, Ferri E, Moscatelli P, Ballarino P, Carpinteri G, Noto P, Gliozzo B, Paladino L, Di Stasio E.

Additive value of blood neutrophil gelatinase-associated lipocalin to clinical judgement in acute kidney injury diagnosis and mortality prediction in patients hospitalized from the emergency department. *Crit. Care* 2013;17:R29.

[47] Haase-Fielitz A, Haase M, Devarajan P. NGAL as a Biomarker of Acute Kidney Injury – A Critical Evaluation of Current Status. *Ann. Biochem. Rev.* 2014 (in press).

[48] Kümpers P, Hafer C, Lukasz A, Lichtinghagen R, Brand K, Fliser D, Faulhaber-Walter R, Kielstein JT. Serum neutrophil gelatinase-associated lipocalin at inception of renal replacement therapy predicts survival in critically ill patients with acute kidney injury. *Crit. Care* 2010;14:R9.

In: Neutrophil Gelatinase-Associated Lipocalin   ISBN: 978-1-63117-984-6
Editors: M. Hur and S. Di Somma   © 2014 Nova Science Publishers, Inc.

Chapter 20

Multi-Markers Approach Including NGAL and other Biomarkers

Salvatore Di Somma[1,], Laura Magrini[1], Benedetta De Berardinis[1] and Mina Hur[2]*

[1]Department of Medical-Surgery Sciences and Translational
Medicine, University Sapienza Rome, Emergency Department
Emergency Medicine Sant'Andrea Hospital, Rome, Italy
[2]Department of Laboratory Medicine, Konkuk
University School of Medicine, Seoul, Korea

Abstract

Acute kidney injury (AKI) is considered an abrupt failure in kidney function. Its assessment relies on diagnostic criteria on the basis of serial measurements of serum creatinine and urine output, that are not sensitive enough for an early diagnosis of AKI.

Recently, in acute pathologic conditions, new biomarkers more sensitive for diagnosing AKI have been developed. Among the new bio-markers: neutrophil gelatinase-associated lipocalin (NGAL), cystatin C, interleukin-18 (IL-18), procalcitonin (PCT), and natriuretic peptides

---

[*]Correspondence: salvatore.disomma@uniroma1.it.

could represent the more suitable ones to be used in a multi-marker approach, especially in an acute setting for critical diseases.

Introduction

Acute kidney injury (AKI) is characterized by functional and structural changes in the kidney and is linked to worse clinical outcomes. Risk, Injury, Failure, Loss, and End-Stage Kidney Disease (RIFLE) and Acute Kidney Injury Network (AKIN) criteria are the most frequently used scoring systems for the detection of AKI [1, 2]. The diagnosis of AKI is, however, often difficult because these criteria and conventional biomarkers such as creatinine and urea are time consuming and, consequently, useless for the early diagnosis of AKI. In the past few years, a growing interest has emerged around the search and validation of new biomarkers more specific and sensitive for AKI diagnosis.

These biomarkers should represent a more precise tool for the diagnosis of AKI and could reasonably improve the sensitivity, specificity, and time for diagnosing AKI. Biomarkers could also help in risk stratification and provide prognostic information on predicting recovery of renal function. For this purpose, cystatin C, kidney injury molecule-1 (KIM-1), Interleukin-18 (IL-18), and NGAL are the most frequently used markers, alone or in combination [3-6]. Among these biomarkers, NGAL has the more robust literature evidences on diagnostic and prognostic powers for AKI [3-8]. Nevertheless, the usefulness of employing more than one biomarker simultaneously could help and ameliorate the assessment of AKI in different critical conditions.

NGAL in Combination with other Biomarkers of AKI

There are very few data in literature addressing the utility of combined use of more than one biomarker in diagnosis and prognosis of AKI. The TRIBE study evaluated more than 100 patients undergoing cardiac surgery [3]. In post-surgery patients, urine IL-18 together with urine and plasma NGAL increased and were linked to the demonstration of high predictive value for AKI [3]. Che et al. [4] also used a multimarker panel in order to diagnose AKI in a cohort of patients following cardiac surgery.

They found that NGAL together with IL-18 and cistatin C was able to predict AKI. Moreover, the prediction of AKI was dependent on sampling time, and NGAL had the best predictive time profile among those markers.

Recently, new data have been published on the usefulness of a multi marker approach with serial assessments of urinary NGAL and urinary liver fatty acid binding protein (L-FABP), before, and serially after surgery. Both biomarkers were significantly increased in patients undergoing surgery ($P < 0.05$). Postoperatively, in AKI group, the peak levels of NGAL and L-FABP occurred 12 and 4 h later, respectively. The area under the receiver operating characteristic (ROC) curves (AUC) for NGAL (at 12 h) and for L-FABP (at 4 h) showed that the most predictive model (NGAL at 12 h and L-FABP at 4 h) and the best combination at the same time point (12 h) was 0.83 [5]. Krawczevski et al. [6] performed a study on paediatric patients undergoing cardiac surgery. They found that urine NGAL, IL-18, L-FABP, and KIM-1 were sequentially predictive biomarkers for AKI and correlated with disease severity and clinical outcomes.

Other studies in several pathological conditions, such as diabetes mellitus [7] and ischemic cardiomyopathy [8], showed the utility of combined NGAL and cystatin C in detecting kidney injury.

In patients with ischemic cardiomyopathy, it has been shown that cystatin C and NGAL serially measured before, and after percutaneous coronary intervention were both strong predictors of death in patients with stable angina, and urinary NGAL was the strongest one [8]. It seems that the combination of kidney functional and damage biomarkers could provide an early and sensitive method to stratify patients with AKI. Han et al. [9] suggested that a multi-marker approach including NGAL could be useful in detecting AKI early after cardiac surgery. Moreover, Haase et al. [10] showed that NGAL in combination with cystatin C correlated with AKI duration after cardiac surgery, and both markers also correlated with the length of stay in intensive care unit after surgery.

NGAL and other Biomarkers in Acute Critical Conditions

Recently, a large interest has been grown in the usefulness of combination of biomarkers for AKI diagnosis in acute illnesses, such as sepsis or acute heart failure (AHF). In patients with suspected sepsis, Kim et al. [11] very recently stressed the importance of measuring simultaneously PCT and NGAL.

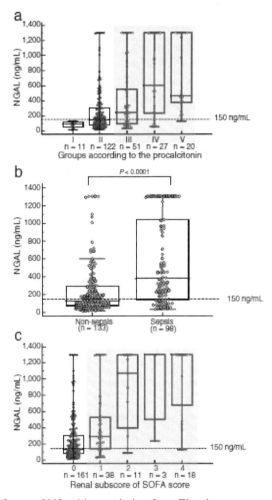

Adapted from reference [11], with permission from Elsevier.

Figure 1. Comparison of NGAL between the PCT groups and the renal subscore of sepsis-related organ failure assessment (SOFA) score: a) the median values of NGAL were all above the medical decision point in septic patients; b) NGAL was significantly higher in septic patients (group III - V) than in non-septic patients (group I - II); c) the median value of NGAL were all above the medical decision point in the groups with renal failure. NGAL was significantly associated with the renal subscore of SOFA score ($P < 0.0001$).

In that study, PCT demonstrated itself being able to correlate with the diagnosis of sepsis, and NGAL was, at the same time, highly sensitive in predicting AKI in the septic patients (Figure 1).

As a consequence, it seems that these two biomarkers could be used together in patients with sepsis in order to diagnose AKI [11].

In another study on septic patients in intensive care unit (ICU), Lentini et al. [12] demonstrated the usefulness of combining NGAL and BNP evaluations together with advanced oxidation protein products (AOPP).

The levels of NGAL, BNP, and AOPP were significantly higher among septic patients compared with non-septic subjects. Among the septic patients, subjects who developed AKI showed significantly higher levels of NGAL, AOPP, and BNP. The correlation among the increases of NGAL, BNP, and AOPP indicated multiorgan involvements in these two conditions of sepsis and AKI [12].

Martensson et al. [13] showed that NGAL, both urinary and plasma, if measured within a pool of other biomarkers, such as PCT, C-reactive protein, and others, was able to predict AKI, but urinary NGAL was more useful. They also demonstrated that elevated plasma NGAL levels were associated with sepsis, independentlyfrom the degree of acute renal dysfunction. A cut-off value 98 ng/mL of NGAL distinguished sepsis from systemic inflammation with high sensitivity (0.77) and specificity (0.79). This suggests that plasma NGAL not only could be the sign of kidney damage but also could help clinicians to identify bacterial infections in critically ill patients [14].

Aydoğdu et al. [15] confirmed the results of Martensson et al. [13]: they showed that plasma NGAL increases in patients with sepsis even in the absence of AKI and suggested that NGAL should be used with caution as a marker of AKI in septic patients. In their study, both plasma and urine cystatin C worked very well for the diagnosis of AKI (AUC 0.82 and 0.86, respectively) in critically ill septic patients. Plasma NGAL performed less well (AUC 0.44), while urinary NGAL showed a significant discrimination for AKI diagnosis (AUC 0.80) [15]. In the GALLANT study, the patients with AHF had the worst outcomes, when both plasma NGAL and BNP levels were high [16]. Patients with high NGAL and low BNP levels also had significantly worse outcomes compared with the other groups where BNP was high and NGAL was low or when both markers were low. The study concluded that the combination of BNP and NGAL tests in heart failure patients at discharge results in a better risk stratification for patients' death and rehospitalization allowing for management decisions with the aim to preserve renal function and to prevent subsequent heart failure-related events [16].

The combination of NGAL with NT pro-BNP has been studied, but only few data are present in literature, which was focused on chronic illnesses about the relevance of hemodynamic and renal changes in ductus arteriosus in preterm babies [17] and in patients with diabetes and proteinuria in chronic heart failure [18].

Our group also proposed a multimarker approach to investigate the presence of AKI in cardio-renal syndromes (CRS) in an emergency setting, using NGAL and BNP simultaneously [19]. Alvelos et al. [20] investigated the performance of NGAL and cystatin C in the early detection of type 1 CRS in patients with AHF. They found a connection between NGAL and type 1 CRS, confirming the utility of NGAL in the early recognition of CRS.

A cutoff value of 170 ng/L was able to predict renal insufficiency in patients with preserved renal function at admission [20].

Conclusion

In different settings of acute pathologic conditions, such as sepsis and AHF, a multimarker approach including NGAL could better define not only diagnosis but also prognosis of AKI patients.

In these diseases, repeated measurements of biomarkers could identify functional and damage changes simultaneously and could also help establish threshold of each biomarker, which could be specific for early signs of organ damage.

References

[1]   Bellomo R, Ronco C, Kellum JA, Mehta RL, Palevsky P, and the ADQI workgroup. Acute renal failure – definition, outcome measu-res, animalmodels, fluid therapy and information technology needs: the Second International Consensus Conference of the Acute Dialysis Quality Initiative (ADQI) Group. *Crit. Care* 2004;8:R204-12.

[2]   Mehta RL, Kellum JA, Shah SV, Molitoris BA, Ronco C, Warnock DG, Levin A, Acute Kidney Injury Network. Acute Kidney Injury Network: report of an initiative to improve outcomes in acute kidney injury. *Crit. Care* 2007;11:R31.

[3]   Parikh CR, Devarajan P, Zappitelli M, Sint K, Thiessen-Phil brook H, Li S, Kim RW, Koyner JL, Coca SG, Edelstein CL, Shlipak MG, Garg AX, Krawczeski CD. TRIBE-AKI Consortium. Postoperative biomarkers predict acute kidney injury and poor outcomes after pediatric cardiac surgery. *J. Am. Soc. Nephrol.* 2011;22:1737–47.

[4]   Che M, Xie B, Xue S, Dai H, Qian J, Ni Z, Axelsson J, Yan. Clinical usefulness of novel biomarkers for the detection of acute kidney injury following elective cardiac surgery. *Nephron. Clin. Pract.* 2010; 115:c66–c72.

[5]   Zeng XF, Li JM, Tan Y, Wang ZF, He Y, Chang J, Zhang H, Zhao H, Bai X, Xie F, Sun J, Zhang Y. Performance of urinary NGAL and L-FABP in predicting acute kidney injury and subsequent renal recovery: a cohort study based on major surgeries. *Clin. Chem. Lab. Med.* 2013

[6]   Krawczeski CD, Goldstein SL, Woo JG, Wang Y, Piyaphanee N, Ma Q, Bennett M, Devarajan P. Temporal relationship and predictive value of urinary acute kidney injury biomarkers after pediatric cardiopulmonary bypass. *JACC* 2011;58:2301-09.

[7]   Assal HS, Tawfeek S, Rasheed EA, El-Lebedy D, Thabet EH. Serum cystatin C and tubular urinary enzymes as biomarkers of renal dysfunction in type 2 diabetes mellitus. *Clin. Med. Insights Endocrinol. Diabetes* 2013;6:7-13.

[8]   Bachorzewska-Gajewskaa H, Tomaszuk-Kazberukc A, Jarockab I, Mlodawskaa E, Lopatowskaa P, Zalewska-Adamieca M, Dobrzycki S, Musial WJ, Malyszko J. Does neutrophil gelatinase-asociated lipocalin have prognostic value in patients with stable angina undergoing elective PCI? A 3-year follow-up study. *Kidney Blood Press. Res.* 2013; 37:280-85.

[9]   Han WK, Wagener G, Zhu Y, Wang S, Lee HT. Urinary bio-markers in the early detection of acute kidney injury after cardiac surge-ry. *Clin. J. Am. Soc. Nephrol.* 2009;4:873-82.

[10]   Haase M, Bellomo R, Devarajan P, Ma Q, Bennett MR, Möckel M, Matalanis G, Dragun D, Haase-Fielitz A. Novel biomarkers early predict the severity of acute kidney injury after cardiac surgery in adults. *Ann. Thorac. Surg.* 2009;88:124-30.

[11]   Kim H, Hur M, Cruz DN, Moon HW, Yun YM. Plasma neutrophil gelatinase-associated lipocalin as a biomarker for acute kidney injury in critically ill patients with suspected sepsis. *Clin. Bio-chem.* 2013;46:1414-18.

[12] Lentini P, de Cal M, Clementi A, D'Angelo A, Ronco C. Sepsis and AKI in ICU patients: the role of plasma biomarkers. *Crit. Care Res. Pract.* 2012;2012:856401.

[13] Martensson J, Bell M, Oldner A, Xu S, Venge P, Martling CR. Neutrophil gelatinase-associated lipocalin in adult septic patients with and without acute kidney injury. *Intensive Care Med.* 2010;36:1333–40.

[14] Martensson J, Bell M, Xu S, Bottai M, Ravn B, Venge P, Martling CR. Association of plasma neutrophil gelatinase-associated lipocalin (NGAL) with sepsis and acute kidney dysfunction. *Biomarkers* 2013;18:349–56.

[15] Aydoğdu M, Gürsel G, Sancak B, Yeni S, Sarı G, Taşyürek S, Türk M, Yüksel S, Senes M, Ozis TN. The use of plasma and urine neutrophilgelatinase associated lipocalin (NGAL) and Cystatin C in early diagnosis of septic acutekidney injury in critically ill patients. *Dis. Markers* 2013;34:237-46.

[16] Maisel AS, Mueller C, Fitzgerald R, Brikhan R, Hiestand BC, Iqbal N, Clopton P, van Veldhuisen DJ. Prognostic utility of plasma neutrophil gelatinase associated lipocalin in patients with acute heart failure: The NGAL EvaLuation Along with B-type NaTriuretic Peptide in acutely decompensated heart failure (GALLANT) trial. *Eur. J. Heart Fail.* 2011;13:846–51.

[17] Tosse V, Pillekamp F, Verde P, Hadzik B, Sabir H, Mayatepek E, Hoehn T. Urinary NT-proBNP, NGAL, and H-FABP may predict hemodynamic relevance of patent ductus arteriosus in very low birth weight infants. *Neonatology* 2012;101:260–66.

[18] Taskapan H, Taskapan MC, Orman I, Ulutas O, Yigit A, Ozyalin F, Yologlu S. NGAL and NT-proBNP levels in diabetic patients with macroproteinuria. *Ren. Fail.* 2013;35:1273-7.

[19] Di Somma S, Gori CS, Salvatori E. How to manage cardiorenal syndromes in the emergency room. *Contrib. Nephrol.* 2010;165:93-100.

[20] Alvelos M, Pimentel R, Pinho E, Gomes A, Lourenço P, Teles MJ, Almeida P, Guimarães JT, Bettencourt. Neutrophil gelatinase-associated lipocalin in the diagnosis of type 1 cardio-renal syndrome in the general ward. *Clin. J. Am. Soc. Nephrol.* 2011;6:476-81.

Index